Better HEALTH™ for You

Denis Toovey

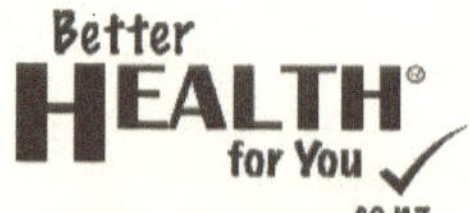

42 Donnington Place,
Sterling Gate, Tauranga, New Zealand. 3110

Disclaimer

ACKNOWLEDGEMENTS

I am grateful for the people who aided and encouraged me: Jenny Argante, John Arts, Sylvia and John Bowden, George Bryant, Jennifer Butler, David Coory, Robert and Bernadette Dee, Chad Dick, Tony Donnelly, Kerin Freeman, Dr Mike Godfrey, Cheryl Goodwin, Eddie and Bev Guddop, Marielle Haringa, Andrew Killick, Wiremu Matthews, Tami Norman, Sue Page, Dr Janice Priest, Karolyn Timarkos, Michelle Triggs, Dr Ted Walford, David Walpole, other colleagues; and, in particular, friends and family.

DEDICATION

Firstly, I dedicate this book to the late Dr David Higgins, who opened my mind to wholistic 'whole/big picture' health when he solved a major medical problem my regular GP could not. Without him, it is unlikely I would ever have written *Better Health for You.*

I also dedicate this book to my wife Judy, who urged me to consult David and who has been an incredible backstop over many years and to our wonderful family, including our six grandchildren.

Last, but not least, I dedicate it, with grateful thanks, to the patients whose stories I share.

Contents

HOW THIS BOOK WILL BENEFIT YOU

Mahatma Gandhi once said, "Health is real wealth, not gold and silver" and Dr Andrew Moulden, US physician and neuroscientist in the USA, says, "Changing the medical system to help people help themselves is the most important work we can do."

With these thoughts in mind and cognisant of the fact that many people around the world suffer or die prematurely from preventable diseases, I have set down my observations and research findings for you. My primary aim is to stop you falling through cracks in the health system by helping you navigate through the maze of confusion and mixed messages.

Health is your most valuable asset. If you want to increase your chances of living a longer, healthier life by seeing the 'big picture' including how to get the best from your lifestyle, health professionals and their treatments, this book is for you.

TESTIMONIAL

"This is an important book by a pharmacist who became increasingly concerned at the limitations and adverse side-effects of medicines.

Fortunately, Denis Toovey had not only sufficient curiosity to look outside the square, but also the courage to act. This book is the result of many years searching for potentially better ways to maintain health in an environment that has become progressively more toxic.

The reader will find answers to many health questions with good evidence-based remedial suggestions. At the very least it ought to be in every library."

Dr Mike Godfrey MBBS.

A number of years ago I was seriously unwell for several months. My doctor diagnosed Chronic Fatigue Syndrome (CFS) and said there was not much he could do for me. As luck would have it, my wife suggested I go to a doctor I met when I was a pharmacist, visiting doctors to advise on cost effective use of medicines. Dr Higgins was unusual in that he focused on nutrition and lifestyle before resorting to medicines. During my visit he checked me out in the orthodox manner and found nothing unusual.

He then enquired if I was open-minded. Not appreciating what he meant, I stated that I was struggling with poor health and desperate for answers. He then proceeded to do some muscle testing, called applied kinesiology that showed my body to be low in boron, zinc and co-enzyme Q10 and not suffering from CFS. After taking supplements to correct the deficiencies, unbelievably, I was back to my normal self within a week.

While I cannot prove Dr Higgins's treatment cured me, this experience opened my mind to the importance of getting an accurate diagnosis, then dealing with the cause(s) - by standing back to look at the 'big picture'. It had taken a crisis to move me to action, which is so often the case for most of us. Dr Higgins became my regular doctor, but was tragically killed in a hit and run incident some years later. Sadly, I have never been able to find a replacement quite like him.

Throughout this book I have used the term 'wholistic' to emphasise a focus on the benefits of a whole 'big picture' approach. This includes holistic (complementary and alternative medicine, focused on dealing with causes of disease), combined with orthodox medicine. *Integrative* and *functional* medicine are alternate terms.

Some years ago in Tauranga I gave a talk on health to a group called 'Recycled Teenagers.' Questions at the end continued for over an hour, revealing a hunger for information, especially in a relaxed setting where some of those listening might hear answers to questions they were afraid to ask. This, and the experience with Dr Higgins and the 'case studies' that follow prompted me to extend my research, find further examples of 'better health' and share that knowledge with others.

In 2007 the World Cancer Research Fund reported a link between obesity and cancer with the consumption of red and processed meat. It recommended that we limit red meat to 500 gram (g) per week (in three to four servings) and minimise the use of processed meats such as sausages and bacon, especially those containing nitrites. A Harvard University study confirmed these findings in 2012.[1] Interestingly, a reporter (probably with little training in health studies) suggested we ignore this information and 'just enjoy life.'

In 2012 two Auckland doctors, whose work had a strong emphasis on nutrition and lifestyle, featured in a television program, *Is Modern Medicine Killing You?* Keen to get one of them to review my book, I found she was too busy, as the media exposure had led to her waiting list ballooning out to nine months. Interestingly, I am not aware of any outcry about the provocative title, which could suggest some acceptance of its truth.

Congratulations on investing in your health by reading this book. I am confident it will make a real difference. The principles are straightforward but remember, there are no magic bullets and good health is not as simple as many seem to think. My advice is to focus on the 'big picture' which is why I have provided you with a myriad of ideas, and invite you to select whatever applies to you as a unique individual.

Think of the content as a fistful of cash, with each note representing different strategies to improve your health and even save you money and take some pressure off the tax burden. If you heed the key messages and work on the Action Plan provided as an appendix, you will be well on the way to better health, including issues to raise with members of parliament, administrators and professionals.

Some uncommon acronyms used in the text are highlighted in bold font with the relevant letters in bold and underlined.

What is important to you?

Think about why you are reading this book. What frustrates you? Would you like to take more responsibility for your health, but are not sure where to start? Consider the following points to get started:

- Information on what good health is and how to achieve it is critical.
- Time for action is now, not when a medical crisis strikes.
- Suspend any disbelief you may have, until the end.
- Attitude makes a difference, so focus on the positive.
- Big picture thinking is beneficial.
- Open-mindedness and acceptance of change (through new information) is important.
- Unresolved issues will continue until reliable research is completed.
- Twenty-one days, at least, is the time it takes to develop a new habit.
- You know your body better than others do, so be prepared to take a stand when you know something is wrong. Be true to yourself.

- Ownership and taking responsibility is essential for progress. You have a greater stake in your health than others do.
- Unique is what you are. Since one size does not fit all, be wary of vague generalizations that may not apply to you.

Science tells us that when presented with a new idea we typically go through four stages: rejected as crazy or too simple to be true or impractical, a degree of acceptance, acknowledgement that the idea is more important than first thought, and finally acceptance and promotion to others.

On the other hand, research at the University of Michigan in 2006 suggests that some misinformed people, when exposed to corrected facts, stubbornly refused to change their minds. Beware of falling into this trap.

CHAPTER 1

Common Health Issues

Health may be defined as the absence of disease, with the body, mind and spirit in harmony with the world. However you define it, health is our most valuable asset, and new information on it is emerging all the time. For instance, imagine what health practitioners fifty years from now might say about today's methods. Despite the billions of dollars spent on research, including cures for cancer, we hardly know why diseases occur and how we can prevent or cure them. Your health can fail for a variety of reasons, including:

- Infections.
- Autoimmune diseases such as rheumatoid arthritis, where, for unknown reasons, the immune system attacks body cells.
- An inexplicable and uncontrolled growth of cells (cancer)
- A poor diet and lifestyle.
- Unhealthy, absent or damaged genes.
- Environmental issues like toxins, injuries and allergies.

The World Health Organization (WHO) believes that by 2020 two-thirds of global disease will be chronic, and strongly associated with poor diet (especially the consumption of refined, processed foods), low-activity lifestyles, and tobacco.

The Chair of Health Workforce New Zealand tells us New Zealand is heading for a shortage of health workers, which, when combined with the retirement of large numbers of post-Second World War baby boomers, will put real pressure on our health system.

Preventable early death and suffering

Globally, many people suffer or die early from preventable diseases including heart disease, cancer, diabetes, obesity, dementia, glaucoma, macular degeneration, autoimmune diseases and depression.

Wholistic 'whole/big picture' health

Just as Dr Higgins opened my mind to wholistic health, Dr Andrew Weill, MD, a wholistic medical practitioner in the USA [www.drweil.com] has stressed the importance of the mind-body relationship.

"It is unacceptable," he said, "for a health practitioner to tell a patient a problem is in their mind because, for that person, beliefs are an integral part of their condition" e.g. some doctors now acknowledge a person can have pain even when there is no physical evidence according to current medical detection skills.[2]

Also, patient-centred care (PCC) respects patients and involves them in the decision-making process and is becoming more common today. It suggests that healing is an active, co-operative process between a practitioner and patient, while 'treatment' implies little or no patient involvement.

PCC results in better outcomes, fewer medical tests, the closer following of advice and more satisfied patients. Not like the case of a patient told by an arthritis specialist that her doctor had been overdosing her on one of her medicines.

According to Professor Marc Cohen, of the Australasian Integrative Medicine Association, "Ultimately medicine has a single aim - to relieve human suffering. When measured against this benchmark, different therapies are effective or ineffective, rather than 'orthodox' or 'unorthodox.' He suggests a multidisciplinary approach in which healthcare professionals work together for the benefit of their patients and the wider community.

To give you an idea of a 'big picture' approach, consider some ways to treat chronic (ongoing) indigestion or heartburn:

- First we should get a correct diagnosis to exclude serious issues like cancer. Treating symptoms while delaying proper investigation could be dangerous.
- We could then focus on treating symptoms by prescribing a long-term medicine to lower acid levels, even though some medicine may affect nutrition and/or increase the chances of infections, as discussed later.
- We could see whether a lack of acid or digestive enzymes was the cause and recommend supplemental betaine and foods like pineapple or kiwifruit.
- We could alter the diet, e.g. reduce fat, chocolate and alcohol; add zinc, fibre or probiotics; recommend vitamins or check if foods like cabbage, onions, bread, etc., were a cause.
- We could eliminate the bacteria Helicobacter pylori that might be a cause. (Discussed in more detail later.)

An interesting website in development that helps with this 'big picture' approach is www.hyperhealth.com.

Physical resilience

During my pharmacy training, a surgeon highlighted the body's fantastic ability to survive, repair itself and adapt to all sorts of challenges. He stressed that many patients get better without visiting their doctor.

In other words the body often healed itself with the right nutrients, in the right balance, at the right time, usually with a little tender loving care. While some people write off risks like smoking because they know of folk who smoked, yet lived to a ripe old age, the fact is that their lifestyle diet, mental attitude and genetics may have been their redeeming factors.

Nature's ways

Our body is a magnificent machine, regulating and maintaining different functions all on its own. For example, circadian rhythms are physical, mental and behavioural changes that follow a roughly 24-hour cycle; and partly regulated by the hormone cortisol, which has its own rhythm; and important regulating roles in blood glucose; the immune system; and metabolism of fat, carbohydrate and protein.

While the theory is not totally proven, research suggests certain health processes give better results if carried out at particular times during this cycle, e.g. filling dental cavities, measuring blood pressure and weight, eating dinner, exercising, taking medicines and testing for asthma.[3] Disruptions of this biorhythm through jet lag and shift work may affect our health.[4]

Nature keeps the body in a state of balance. For instance, our sympathetic nervous system allows us to move quickly in a 'fight or flight' response by speeding up our heart, dilating the pupils of our eyes and sending more blood to skeletal muscles. Then the para-sympathetic nervous system has an opposing or balancing effect.

In any one day, millions of biological processes take place in our bodies. While errors can occur, the body usually corrects them, as long as it has the necessary nutrients and optimal conditions to do so. Our body will also excrete or conserve nutrients and water according to our intake and need. For example, an increased intake of vitamin C leads to increased excretion, yet, over time, increased absorption.[5]

Just because something is natural, it isn't necessarily good for us. There are natural poisons such as curare, and some fat-soluble vitamins may accumulate in our fat stores to a toxic level. For many nutrients and medicines, a delicate balance exists between what is and isn't useful e.g. the trace mineral selenium has many roles and benefits (discussed later), but too much of it can be toxic. So we have blood tests to ensure safe body levels.

Ageing

Living a long, disease-free life and dying peacefully in our sleep is the goal of most of us. Typically infectious diseases and acute illnesses, once the leading cause of death, have given way to degenerative illnesses that people may live with for decades. The book *Heathcheque* by Morgan and Simmons found that half of the people in the UK had a chronic medical condition, with half having more than one disease, referred to as 'co-morbidity.'

Telomeres are part of the DNA (deoxyribonucleic acid) in chromosomes that protect the ends from deterioration, or from rearranging with each other. Think of it like the plastic ends we place on shoelaces to stop them unravelling. According to Hayflick's Theory, as we get older, telomeres shorten with each cell division, reducing the life of those cells, so they eventually die. Good nutrition repairs this shortening.

Scientists are looking at cancer cells that display the opposite effect, to find ways of slowing ageing. Products like TA65, from the herb astralagus, look promising, with research continuing.[6] A medical test in Canada looks at the length of the telomeres to give an idea of how many years of life one had left (if one wanted to know).

Dr Oz, a heart surgeon in the USA featured ageing on one of his television shows. [www.doctoroz.com] He commented how skin provides a window to health, as evidenced by the skin damage shown by smokers. Dr Oz warned about concealing the tell-tale signs by covering the skin with cosmetics when visiting doctors. Look for clues to ageing, such as eyelids drooping to touch your upper eyelashes. Or pinch and release your lower eyelid to see if it takes more than two seconds to return to normal. In addition, look for uneven skin colouring, smile and frown creases, and stress lines on the forehead.

Wrinkles can be a reflection of yo-yo diets, where the skin stretches with weight gain and does not retract with subsequent weight loss. Beauty treatment for the skin is mostly about moisturisers and sun protection, so beware of unproven, expensive products.

Why are we living longer?

The average life expectancy at birth was 25 years in 1800 and 50 years in 1900. Today in New Zealand it is 79 years for men and 83 for women, with the gap narrowing. Some suggest a high infant mortality rates skewed earlier figures, and that people living beyond fifteen often lived to see their grandchildren.[7] So it seems decreased infant mortality brought about by improved housing, hygiene, vaccines, antibiotics and medicines has played a significant role in longevity.

Nutrition plays a key role both positively and negatively, as we shall see, and research suggests that the longer you live, the longer you are likely to live.[8] Some now suggest 60 is 'middle age' and 90 is 'old age.' The proportion of older people in New Zealand is steadily increasing, due to a falling birth rate and the bubble of baby boomers who were born between 1946 and 1964. By the year 2036, 40% of the population will be over 65.[9] Interestingly, Japan has more than 30,000 residents over the age of one hundred — the highest rate per capita in the world.

The *Life and Living in Advanced Age* (LILAC) study in New Zealand aims to get greater insight into why some people live longer.[10] In his book *Blue Zones*, Dan Buettner suggests we are living longer, partly because of our genes (20%) but mostly through an improved lifestyle.[11] He looked at parts of the world where people were living longer and healthier lives and found areas like Icaria in Greece where the average lifespan was 90. The lifestyle of the people included a special honey and tea, daytime naps, little meat, lots of beans, nuts and vegetables, and walking.

A study of a population of Italian heritage in the Rosetto region in Pennsylvania, USA, found longevity and good health associated with a strong sense of community interaction. Researchers have also found populations in parts of the world with virtually no heart disease, as we shall see in the food section.

CHAPTER 2

Fact or Fiction?

Sometimes we read a story in a magazine or hear something that seems to make sense at the time. Later, when we get a different angle on the subject, we realise we didn't know what we thought we knew.

When patients visiting our pharmacy claimed their treatment hadn't worked, we often found they had come to the wrong conclusion. Some had not given enough time for medicines to work; others had difficulty understanding that the treatment might have slowed the progression of their condition; still others overrated their treatment, because of the placebo effect, with its powers of suggestion.

Some put a result down to coincidence, and some were going to get better anyway. Since information in isolation can be misleading, we need to step back and consider the big picture including context, validity of information, alternative points of view and individual variability.

In today's world, some people appear to think it is all right to believe and say whatever they want, even if there is no scientific evidence to support it. Thus many people believed a story reported by www.hoax-slayer.com about an egg cooking when placed between two cell phones. Clearly, we often need to do some research before adding information to our 'knowledge bank.'

While some say science can be isolated from the everyday world, arrogant in its claims, and patronising in how it presents information, it plays an important role in knowledge we cannot ignore.

Scientific principles

A Scots doctor, James Lind (1716-1794), was possibly the first person to conduct a scientific health experiment to demonstrate that fruit and vegetables containing vitamin C prevented the disease, scurvy, unlike cats and dogs that produce their own.

First he had an idea (theory) that food might be the cause of the problem. Then he worked out a way to test his idea by giving different foods to different groups of people. From this he got results (data) that enabled him to draw conclusions i.e. he used a systematic approach to prove a theory.

Statistics

We often joke that those who use statistics are able to interpret figures (data) to mean whatever they want them to. Statistics can be notoriously slippery, misused by the unscrupulous or misinterpreted by the unwary. For instance, a counsellor once told me the standard questionnaire used by the bureaucracy to diagnose depression was too simplistic to be statistically reliable.

In *Calculated Risks: How to Know When Numbers Deceive You*, 48 experienced doctors were placed into two groups and given information about a cancer-screening test. They were then asked to give the probability that a person who tested positive actually had the disease. The first group received information in the conventional mathematical way (conditional probability), with many getting the answer wrong. The second group received the information in a 'user-friendly whole number' format, and most arrived at the correct answer.

In another example, when patients were told there was a 30% chance of experiencing sexual dysfunction with a medicine, most interpreted this to mean there would be a problem 30% of the time. When told three out of ten users would experience a problem, they easily and accurately understood the intended meaning.

When interpreting data, it is important to differentiate between the average (total divided by the number of items), the median (mid-point) and the mode (most frequent) to ensure any skewing is accounted for. For example, a group of health-conscious people who are living longer may distort the average upwards, in which case the median is more appropriate.

Probability counts for nothing, if you happen to be the statistic. The incidence of a disease might be one in a thousand but 100% if it is you.

Medical research

Often the benefits of medical treatments are not dramatic. Sometimes they just outweigh the risks, i.e. more about shades of grey than about black or white. This is why guarantees are usually not given. Because it is hard to eliminate external influences, most treatments require careful science, combined with reliable statistical analysis to see if they offer significant benefit. To give you an appreciation of the complexity of the process, consider the following:

- Most studies require a great deal of planning, staff, time, patients and money.

- There must be clarity about what is measured, in whom and how. Comparisons must be logical, i.e. similar products in comparable doses.

- Participants should be adequately informed about risks and benefits associated with a study. This is commonly referred to as 'informed consent.'

- Reliability of memory and ability to complete questionnaires are important.

- Is the trial double blind, so that no one directly involved in the study knows who is on the placebo, and who is on the real treatment? This is designed to counter the placebo effect that has been shown to be high in some studies. We also need to be sure patients who might be more susceptible to the placebo effect are not 'selected out' from a study.

- Is the study controlled? Is a treated group compared with a similar group of people on placebo, (treatment that appears to be the same, but has no activity)? Not knowing whether or not any individual is on the real medicine reduces the factors that could distort the results. An example was a study of the benefits of fish oil on school performance. This was all done at the same school and students shared information, meaning the results were unreliable.[12]

- Is the study randomised? Are people assigned to groups randomly to eliminate experimenter influence? For example, people call a phone number and a computer allocates a random number.

- Are there enough people in the groups to eliminate chance outcomes?

- Are results published in a reputable, peer-reviewed journal without financial benefits that could compromise standards?

- Does a drug company produce publications deliberately put together to resemble peer-reviewed journals (and can therefore mislead readers?)

- Research that is negative about a product may never be published and remain in the bowels of some laboratory.

- An article in the *New Scientist* says, "It is time medical journals stopped behaving like a medieval church, with the opinion that only scholars will be reading their content. Moreover, they should be presented so as to be useful to readers with an interest in, but little technical knowledge of, a subject."[13]

- Dr Lind died 40 years after publishing his research on vitamin C, at a time when some professionals still did not believe it. Similarly, some doctors were slow to accept the idea that microbes (germs, bacteria, etc.) caused infectious diseases.

- The sophistication of evidence increases as follows: expert opinion, small non-randomized trials, small, randomised controlled trials and large, statistically significant, double blind crossover, randomly controlled trials (RCT). Following a number of trials a review, using a mathematical tool called a meta-analysis, is used to assess the overall picture.

Considering the issues above, it is easy to see how new research information can be a long time coming into the public domain. It may even be out of date by the time it gets to us.

Drug companies are further discussed in the section on medicines, but for now some suggestions for the regulation of medical research include the following raised in *The Truth about Drug Companies*, written by Dr M. Angell:

- We need to strengthen regulatory bodies in some countries.
- Drug companies should not control all their clinical testing.
- Shortened patent periods may sometimes be appropriate.
- The prices of medicines should be reasonable and uniform.

Pragmatic clinical trials

Patients are more likely to adhere to treatment if they are involved in controlled clinical trials.[14] Furthermore, most studies compare a medicine against a placebo, which does not provide much help for doctors wanting to know the best treatment for a particular patient with a number of diseases who is taking a variety of medicines. Because of these limitations, we are seeing the emergence of 'pragmatic' clinical trials, focused on information based on real-life situations, e.g. comparisons of clinically-relevant interventions from a diverse range of doctors with a diverse range of patients. While designed to reflect 'real world' clinical practice, these studies have their limitations.

The Information Age

It is said that many people now refer to Internet health websites before consulting health professionals. This reflects the move from the industrial age to the information age. Beware of people with little or no knowledge (or guarantee) about health products they're selling.

Internet services can be powerful and helpful, as seen in a 2011 story about a mother who put a photo of her ill child on Facebook, where two paediatricians suggested the problem was Kawasaki Disease, a rare autoimmune condition. Lauding the process, the doctor treating the child, made a quick diagnosis.[15]

Most of us believe we cannot have too much information. Yet research suggests there are times when it complicates situations, leaving us in a state of 'paralysis by analysis.' Malcolm Gladwell gives an example of this in his book *Blink*. He writes of a cardiologist at a Chicago hospital who eventually persuades accident and emergency doctors to focus on three symptoms to decide if chest-pain patients need admitting to the expensive heart unit, rather than the general medical ward.[16]

While much good information is available on the Internet, be wary as it is not policed, so inaccurate information can prevail. When this is added to a lack of understanding of specialist subjects, people may take inappropriate action or endure unnecessary anxiety and end up in a group commonly referred to as the 'worried well.'

When using the Internet, take care you're not acting upon superseded information. Start by checking dates of publication and look at reputable sites recommended by reliable sources, including articles in quality, scientific journals. Be sure to research the big picture, as most orthodox medical websites are likely to ignore natural products or services and vice versa. Websites such as www.wolframalpha.com and www.pingar.com may solve this problem as they aim to provide answers to questions, rather than simply supplying a high number of links to websites, obtained using search engines currently.

Many years ago I was excited to read a story about an American doctor working with a computer expert to put all his medical knowledge onto a database. His mission was to help doctors in the diagnosis and treatment of patients. Just as farmers use GPS tracking to take the guesswork out of spreading fertiliser and hospitals introduce electronic prescribing systems to reduce medication errors and save time, we are likely to see computers play a greater role to ensure optimal, up-to-date care is delivered to patients.

Absence of evidence is not evidence of absence

Writer Upton Sinclair once said, "In some cases research will not be done, because it is difficult to get a man to understand something when his salary depends on not understanding it."

Other reasons why research is not undertaken include a lack of interest or finance, low profit potential, ignorance of the relevance of an observation, and a perception that science tends not to favour models that do not fit with established theories.

Common sense

Sometimes we go overboard trying to prove things that are too difficult, too costly or too impractical, when common sense (that has assisted human survival over centuries) has a role to play. For instance conducting a double-blind trial on parachutes would be an oxymoron. Common sense does not get the recognition it deserves, as aptly summed up in an 'obituary' printed in the *London Times*:

> *"Today we mourn the passing of a beloved old friend, Common sense, who has been with us for many years. No one knows how old he was, since his birth records were long ago lost in bureaucratic red tape. He reminds us of such valuable lessons as knowing when to come in out of the rain, why the early bird gets the worm, and that life is not always fair and that maybe it was my fault. Common sense lived by simple, sound financial policies such as 'Do not spend more than you earn' and 'Adults, not children, are in charge.'*
>
> *"His health began to deteriorate rapidly when well-intentioned, overbearing regulations were set in place. Reports of a six-year-old boy charged with sexual harassment for kissing a classmate and a teacher fired for reprimanding an unruly student worsened his condition. Common sense lost ground when parents attacked teachers for doing the job that the parents had failed to do, i.e. disciplining unruly children. It declined even further when schools were required to get parental consent to administer sun lotion, but could not inform parents when a student became pregnant and wanted an abortion.*
>
> *"Common sense lost the will to live as criminals received better treatment than their victims and you could not defend yourself from a burglar in your own home, or the burglar could sue you for assault. Common sense finally gave up the will to live, after a woman failed to realize that a steaming cup of coffee was hot. After she spilled some on her lap, she received a huge settlement.*
>
> *"Common sense was preceded (in death) by his parents, Truth and Trust, his wife Discretion, his daughter Responsibility and his son Reason. Four stepbrothers survive him: I Know my Rights, I Want it Now, Someone Else is to Blame and I am a Victim. Not many attended his funeral, because so few realized he was gone."*

In 2011 a report suggested blackberries reduced asthma. Without being too facetious, some would suggest a need to research it, as a team, working under the supervision of a person of superior intellect, paid for their time.

The research would then need to be published in medical jargon (more on this later), employing politically correct gender-neutral terms and long words. It would then be peer-reviewed, making it likely to be rejected if it went against the wisdom of the time, as the expert reviewer would by definition be someone who believed the ruling myth of the day.

Once past this hurdle, and especially if published in a journal of repute - do not ever refer to these as 'magazines' - it would then be acceptable for the conclusions to be extrapolated, far beyond the evidence. Common sense tells us that if blackberries help, then great.

Be careful though, as advice that seems to make sense can be misleading. An article in a women's magazine featured a chef who suggested it was an urban myth that if live mussels didn't open when cooked they were unsafe. "As long as they smell fresh they are okay," he said. Because of the risk of contracting food poisoning, rather than blindly following this advice, look for evidence to back his claim, which was missing from the article.

Common sense and gut-feeling do play a part, but because some things may not be as they seem, often we need research to confirm or negate our beliefs, e.g. brown bread may be simply highly-processed coloured bread.

In another example, a news story headlined, 'Running makes you fat' focused on the idea that exercise increases the release of cortisol, which could lead to additional stomach fat. In reality, if we put things into context, we might find the problem was more about people over-estimating the calories burned during exercise, and the amount of food they could subsequently eat. Hence more research could be necessary.

Ask good probing questions

Today there are over 24,000 medical and scientific journals. In light of this, be wary of people making 'statements of fact.' Since nobody can possibly know it all, it's better to use expressions such as 'there is a high/low probability of...' or 'as far as I know...' when sharing information.

I trust by now you appreciate the importance of reliable health information. So if I asked you if eggs were good for you, what would you say? If you answered yes or no, you would have fallen into a common trap, as more information is required. Just as a good scientist would suggest, "It depends," so you need to drill down into the subject.

Ask good, probing and open-ended questions such as, "Where did the eggs come from? How fresh are they and how were they cooked?" Although eggs are a good source of nutrients and contain relatively high amounts of cholesterol, for most people only a small amount goes into the blood, so are fine, up to one per day, so long as intake of other saturated fats are low.

Experiment and learn

Experience comes from doing things to gauge the results (experimenting) and learning from those experiences, so as not to repeat mistakes or 'reinvent the wheel.' A recipe tells us what to do, but experience fills in any gaps in that information, such as how finely we need to cut the onions and how quickly we need to cook them.

On your journey to better health, experiment with new ideas and do not be put off by answers that seem too simple or too good to be true. Remember, too, that you need to keep doing something for at least three to six weeks for it to become a habit. Only then can you properly test its validity.

We all display different levels of ability, ranging from knowing we don't know anything about a subject (conscious incompetence) to where we know a little, yet think we know it all (unconscious incompetence), to where we know and do something well (conscious competence).

To improve my lawn bowls, I studied a book on the subject and mentioned this to an expert bowler. His response was, "There's no need to read books. Just get out and do it." A reminder that some people learn by watching and copying, without getting knowledge of techniques etc., first.

Trainee pharmacists complete a four-year degree, after which they have a year working with a mentor pharmacist, to certify competency, matching theory with real-life situations. When mentoring trainees, I always stressed that their degree was only the beginning and that they needed to continue learning and applying new knowledge throughout their professional life.

William Butler Yeats summed this up beautifully when he said, "Education is not the filling of a bucket, but the lighting of a fire." Regarding your health, never stop learning and fully accept that ideas may change with ongoing research.

This desire to remain competent reminds me of the surgeon who always booked a room for an extra day or two after a conference to digest what he had learned there. This is a good practice, as it is so easy to return to a busy workplace and let new ideas fall by the wayside.

Modern education puts greater emphasis on 'self-directed learning,' where individuals use learning methods that suit them. In this scenario, the teacher is the 'guide on the side' or facilitator, not the 'sage on the stage.'

Discoveries and inventions

Science is having a significant impact on medicine, with new information and inventions already here, or waiting around the corner. Some take many years to be available commercially. Medical inventions include robotic and keyhole surgery, lasers to kill nail fungi, pancreatic cells from purebred pigs used for Type 2 diabetics and artificial corneas, to name a few.

Sometimes things are rediscovered, e.g. modified electro-convulsive therapy (ECT) has re-emerged to treat some forms of depression.

With 1.7 million deaths in 2009, tuberculosis is one of the biggest killers in the developing world. If diagnosed early it is curable, and so a new test that is 99% accurate, and makes a diagnosis in 100 minutes, is invaluable, compared with the two months it took for the old test.

It seems about half the population have a gene that makes them happy to take risks, like volunteering as guinea pigs for new research. Unless you are in a desperate situation, like the man with a plastic heart, connected to a pump that he carried around while waiting for a heart transplant, I urge caution when considering new products or services, since adverse effects may take some time to emerge.

Such was the case of the leaking PIP breast implants made from unauthorised, industrial grade chemicals. Originally it was thought they hadn't been used in New Zealand, but two years after a recall was announced in 2010, it turned out that this was not the case. Worse still, there was no system to track affected patients. A UK report in 2012 said the implants had up to six times the rupture rate of normal implants, but the chemicals were not toxic. However, the founder of the company that sold the product is facing criminal charges and a class action against the company is proceeding.

Stem cells

Research into stem cells grew out of findings at the University of Toronto in the 1960s.[17] Defined as biological cells that differentiate into specialised cell types, they can even produce more stem cells. They also act as a repair system for the body, replenishing tissues and maintaining the normal turnover of regenerative organs, such as blood, skin or intestinal tissues.

Research in Germany (led by Professor A. Zeiher) is looking into the use of stem cells to repair a heart muscle, damaged in a heart attack. In another instance, in 2012 a plastic mould of part of a person's airway, coated with their stem cells, replaced a cancerous part, surgically removed.

There is a trend to store young stem cells with long telomeres for use later in life. Key sources are umbilical cords, bone marrow and fat, including younger, close blood relatives. Research in Japan in 2014 has found some mice cells reverted to stem cells on exposure to acid.

CHAPTER 3

How Do You See the World?

Your brain operates within your skull, relying on your senses to provide it with information about the outside world, which determines your worldview (perception of the world). For example, you could be forgiven for not knowing, unless you had been told, that on a calm day the earth is spinning at 1,600km per hour at the equator.

Many factors contribute to our worldview, including parents, friends, culture, teachers, religion, genetics, professionals and the media. In fact, some experts suggest most of our perception and behaviour is set by the time we are eight years old. [18]   If true it emphasises the impact of role models early in life. Indeed, research suggests that the children of parents who regularly buy fruit and vegetables are more willing to eat them.

Your conscious mind decides whether or not you will accept new information. However, your subconscious mind works beneath the surface to absorb information without judgment, including whether or not it is true. You are not conscious of this process, and yet it powerfully affects your behaviour.

Research suggests the brain will even act to help make something you believe come true. This is why surgeon B. Siegel suggests it is not a good idea to limit a patient's vision of what the future holds by telling them they only have a certain amount of life left, or will never achieve full mobility after an operation.

Many years ago I had tightness in my chest, and was anxious I might be having a heart attack. When a doctor diagnosed this as a strained muscle, the tension and tightness disappeared, highlighting, yet again, the power of the mind.

Dr Maxwell Maltz MD, a renowned plastic surgeon, observed that some patients who had facial surgery for disfigurement showed positive changes in self-esteem and personality, yet others did not. He suggests the brains of the latter had not accepted the improvements, demonstrating the power of the mind.[19] Moreover, a *New Scientist* article (2009) showed negative beliefs can have a detrimental effect on the outcome of a heart attack.

Human beings can go through life with beliefs that are real to them, yet are actually false, something akin to an optical illusion. Can you see how complications can arise out of a conflict between perception and reality? For example, a bull gets fat and muscular eating grass, yet some people overlook this fact and think meat is the only source of protein when grains, nuts, seeds, legumes (peas, beans) and some vegetables are all sources.

Don't let negative and false thoughts become self-fulfilling prophecies, and remember the word **fear** is an acronym for **f**alse **e**xpectations **a**ppearing **r**eal. Most of the greatest battles you're ever likely to face are inside your head.

In *The Secret*, Rhonda Byrne suggests people tend to get more of what they focus on. So if a person focuses on their painful arthritic knee, the pain will seem worse. To keep things positive, think challenges (not problems) and eliminate words like 'try,' as it implies you will just 'have a go,' and the results don't matter. It is far better to say what you intend to do and then do it.

Confusion and misinformation

The film *Erin Brockovich* tells the story of the toxicity of hexavalent chromium, also known as chromium-6. Used in leather tanning, electroplating and textile manufacturing, the chemical is associated with cancer in rats and lung cancer in humans, and appeared in some drinking water in the USA.

Initially, many people thought the story was about chromium picolinate, a different form of the mineral, used in food and supplements to aid blood sugar control. This story highlights how easily misinformation can creep into our world.

Understanding the principles of science puts you in a better position to avoid confusion, e.g. many people use the terms *cold*, and the more serious *flu*, interchangeably, yet the symptoms (including headache, fever and aches) and treatments are distinctly different with some symptoms mimicking the gravely serious bacterial meningitis.

Fake aspects of our world

It could be said we're all a bit of a fraud at times as we tend to put on a façade or persona in public and conform to how we think people expect us to behave. An example might be giving our teeth an extra special clean before going to the dentist, hoping it will make up for those times when we were not so conscientious.

When we look at the world around us, some of what we're exposed to is so exaggerated or blatantly false we might even think we're abnormal and that others live in some sort of perfect world.

With all the emphasis on weight reduction today, we need to be wary of the impact this could have on underweight people, especially females with a body mass index (BMI) of less than 18, often associated with serious medical problems like anorexia and bulimia. Whilst research suggests a perfectionist personality plays a role, so too does the fashion industry, with comments like, "Clothes look better on thinner, taller models."

Recognising the problem, Israel will not let anybody with a BMI below 18.5 on a catwalk. Some major magazines have followed this precedent and no longer feature models under sixteen, or with eating disorders.

In another example of this fake world, an advertisement included the term, 'The photo may be dramatized,' which translates to 'The photo has been enhanced.' In 2011 a photographer told me almost all photos in the popular magazines she shoots for are touched up, using computer software, to make the models look better than they really are.

Research at Victoria University in New Zealand found 40% of 11 to 16 year old females were unhappy with their body weight. This presented a major source of anxiety and self-image that could lead to depression and anorexia. The report suggested some of this came from media pressure to conform to certain body ideals that were unrealistic.

Just as a 'behind the scenes' documentary showed three different dogs were used to portray a single dog in a television commercial, it is likely some reality television shows feature exaggerated scenes, stimulated by financial rewards for the participants. This is a reminder to beware of false messages putting undue pressure on you to do things that are not good for your health. Follow Steve Jobs' advice: "Do not live someone else's life."

There are times, however, when you might want to 'fake it until you make it,' e.g. to maintain confidence while losing weight, wear clothes that compliment your shape, rather than accentuate the bulges.

'Normal' behaviour

The documentary *Consumed* discusses man's movement from the hunter-gatherer age to the agricultural age, to the industrial age and so into the information and marketing age. Now that basic needs have been met, sexual attraction, prestige and status from consumerism have become 'the norm.'

Most of us tend to conform to the world around us, e.g. a group of overweight friends taunt a trim member of the group because she does not fit the group norm, and the 'tall poppy brigade' drags achievers down to their level. The impact of the world on our behaviour can be subtle. For example, society tends to associate the word 'drink' with alcohol.

Sometimes we conform without realising it, even in ways that undermine our own values, e.g. a gift of a doll with a feeding bottle, when we acknowledge the value of breast-feeding.

CHAPTER 4

The Media and Advertising

Media refers to the means by which information and entertainment reaches us. It can have a major effect on our worldview, especially through sensationalised headlines and stories that may be long-winded, out of context, incomplete and even untrue.

Take for example a newspaper report in 2010, entitled 'Vitamin pills linked to breast cancer.' Whilst the headline reads as a statement of fact, when the story (and original report) are scrutinised, words and terms emerge such as 'plausible,' 'not statistical' and 'more research needed.' In addition, the absolute risk (actual population figures) meant just two extra deaths per 100, over ten years, might occur.

In a report on the media in the UK covering a week entitled *How far should we trust health reporting?* Dr Ben Goldacre, an epidemiologist (medical doctor who studies the health of populations) found that in 111 claims the vast majority were supported by insufficient evidence, with 10% possible, 12% cent probable and in only 15% was the evidence convincing.[20]

Whilst accepting there are limitations to his work, he concludes, 'this is an interesting finding' and goes on to say 'people who work in public health bend over backwards to disseminate evidence-based information to the public, and wonders if they should also focus on documenting and addressing the harm done by journalists.'

In 2008, a study carried out by a journalist, who now works on quantitative studies of media, found that out of 500 health articles, only 35% were satisfactory.[21] Interestingly, if a study appears in the *New York Times* it is also likely be reported in other papers, according to the *New England Journal of Medicine.*

In 2010, a story in a local newspaper about headaches included the comment 'take a few paracetamol.' Concerned that some people might interpret this as taking more than the recommended dose at a time, I rang the reporter and suggested she get a technical person to scrutinise this type of report before publishing it. I got the feeling she wasn't that keen on my idea.

Whilst reasonably safe at normal doses, paracetamol can be extremely dangerous in the overdose situation, especially if taken with a high intake of alcohol.

With the media tainted by unscrupulous practices like phone hacking, its integrity is certainly in question. To move forward, it must ensure it reports responsibly and does not abuse the basic principle of freedom of the press. In line with this, journalists should provide full details of the source of information, give appropriate prominence to any corrections to articles, and follow up stories thoroughly and in a balanced way.

Advertisements and 'infomercials' are designed to get us to take action and buy the product or service. We need to be wary of the accuracy of material presented to us, i.e. beware of so called 'interviews' espousing the merits of such products and services, with no actual evidence to back up claims.

This is a bit like some health company promotions I have attended that were labelled as 'training sessions,' yet speakers did not take questions from the floor, to ensure integrity and transparency. On one such occasion, a salesman presented the benefits of a cough and cold product to an audience of mainly pharmacy assistants, yet did not mention precautions with the pseudoephedrine in it. Needless to say, I intervened to correct this.

A New Zealand television program in 2011 analysed advertisements for beauty products including one to enhance eyelashes, which gave the impression that the cosmetic was responsible for the results, yet fine print at the bottom of the screen mentioned the use of false eyelashes.

Sometimes advertisements create authority for the product itself, using terms like 'hypo-allergenic, clinically proven and dermatologist-tested' that are totally meaningless, if not legally defined. Be wary of high profile people endorsing products they know little about, yet reap rewards from doing so. It is noteworthy that authorities usually do not take any action, until someone makes a complaint. Given the consequences of misleading information on your health, always ask good probing questions, and check resources to validate information.

Direct to consumer advertising

Some years ago I told a pharmacy patient with osteoporosis (brittle bones) that Pharmac, the District Health Boards' buying agency, had commenced subsidising a medicine that might improve her condition. She asked me how long it had been available in New Zealand.

When I said it was about a year, she further questioned me as to why her doctor had not mentioned it. I suggested either he did not know it was available; or had made the decision that she couldn't afford the monthly private cost of about $100, or he did not think it was suitable for her. She contacted him, and he prescribed the medicine. Her disappointment was evident, as she could afford to pay and had been suffering badly with her condition for a long time.

In another situation, a past associate Minister of Health complained about a drug company advertising a medicine to treat shingles. What he probably did not appreciate was the importance of early diagnosis, as treatment within 72 hours of symptoms, including sharp, stabbing pains on one side of the body, is essential to reduce the risk of lifelong nerve pain, known as 'post-herpetic neuralgia.'

To my mind, publication of this information in widely-read magazines could only be helpful, especially as people may easily let three days lapse before going to a doctor. Even then, the diagnosis might be missed, e.g. I developed pain in my leg and an after-hours doctor diagnosed a hernia. Two days later, my local doctor thought it was a pulled muscle. When a rash arose two days later, the diagnosis was shingles.

These stories are examples of why I believe in direct-to-consumer advertising, so long as it is not promotion of less than ideal medicines like some sleeping pills that could lead to addiction and personality changes.

CHAPTER 5

Risk Factors for Disease

Heart disease is a big killer and in about 30% cent of cases, the first symptom is sudden death. The key here is to appreciate the importance of knowing what factors are increasing your chances of dying early, especially as some diseases brewing in the body show no obvious symptoms, and the benefits of action taken to reduce them may not be immediately apparent.

A heart attack occurs when a blood clot obstructs the flow of blood to a part of the heart's muscle, leading to the death of that part, if not quickly cleared. The severity depends on the amount of muscle affected. It may help to think of the blood vessels in your heart muscle as the branches of a tree, where cutting off a twig would be like suffering a very minor heart attack, and so on.

Be sure to stay up-to-date with symptoms of a heart attack, like chest tightness, and be especially aware that patients might experience different symptoms, including pain in the jaw, neck, stomach or shoulder, nausea, indigestion, shortness of breath, dizziness and unusual fatigue. If in any doubt, phone 111 (New Zealand) to discuss whether an ambulance is needed or not.

If you are a candidate for regular low dose aspirin to reduce heart attacks and strokes, Dr Oz says, take with the evening meal to reduce stomach irritation and to cover the early morning when most heart attacks seem to occur. Interestingly, research suggests skipping breakfast may cause shock and increase the risk of a heart attack. Research at Oxford University (Rothwell) suggests aspirin may also reduce the chances of some cancers metastasizing, i.e. moving to other parts of the body.

A stroke occurs as either a blockage or a bleed from a ruptured blood vessel in the brain. Remember the acronym **FAST** to help you recognise a stroke: i.e. **f**ace (one side droopy), **a**rms (raised, with one side weaker), **s**peech (a simple sentence slurred) and **t**ime lost could be lost brain. [www.stroke.org.nz; www.knowyournumbers.co.nz]

There are up to one hundred risk factors for heart disease and strokes, but most focus on about fifteen. Others are emerging, i.e. links between low birth weight to heart disease and diabetes. Some experts suggest a moderate reduction in a number of risk factors is better than an all-out reduction in a single factor. Now let us take a closer look at some key ones remembering that whilst the focus here is on risk factors for heart attack and stroke, some apply to other diseases.

Erectile dysfunction (impotence)

Studies show around 40% of men over 40 years of age experience some degree of erectile dysfunction (ED). The important point here is that this could be a clue to heart and circulation issues that may need further investigation. The problem is that men generally will not talk about such subjects and tend to go searching for a quick fix.

This reminds me of a study on health advice undertaken some years ago that found some shop assistants, when presented with a problem like ED, focused on selling a remedy rather than referring patients to a doctor for investigation and a proper diagnosis first. The study found pharmacists were extremely good at referring patients to other professionals.

High blood pressure (BP)

As we age, our blood vessels tend to become narrow and hardened, making it harder for the heart to pump blood around our body, resulting in hypertension (jargon for high blood pressure.) Like many risk factors, it is usually present without symptoms.

Cholesterol

Cholesterol is an essential component of cells throughout the body that generates three-quarters of its needs, with the rest coming from food. The U.S. Food and Drug Authority (FDA) recommend a maximum of 300mg per day. Given there is only one form of cholesterol, why do people talk about 'good' and 'bad' cholesterol?

In simple terms, think of the liver as a cholesterol factory where good and bad refers to the 'truck' in which it is carried around the body. 'Bad' LDL (low-density lipoprotein) cholesterol is 'trucked' to blood vessels to repair leaks in blood vessels. Unfortunately, it can also lead to atherosclerosis, jargon for a build-up of fatty plaque in blood vessel walls, obstructing blood flow that may lead to a clot, or even burst. LDL-cholesterol levels link to intake of saturated and trans-fatty acids (TFA), discussed in the food section.

On the other hand, good HDL (high-density lipoprotein) cholesterol is the form being 'trucked' away for excretion. A good way to remember the difference is to think **H** for '**h**ealthy' **H**DL and **L** for '**l**ousy' **L**DL.

Ideas about the role of cholesterol in health began many years ago with a project to study an entire community in the USA, i.e. the city of Framingham. The study made many discoveries, including the fact that those with a higher ratio of total cholesterol to HDL had the greatest risk of a heart attack or stroke. If you think about it, the higher your 'healthy' HDL the better, as this decreases this ratio value. Other tests, including LDL levels, complete the whole picture.

Some professionals suggest the current focus on cholesterol is 'over the top,' as it does not tell how much plaque build-up there is, and that inflammation, sugar and insulin resistance are major risk factors, as we shall see. In *Prevent and Reverse Heart Disease*, author Dr Esselstyn, a surgeon in Cleveland, USA suggests it is the smaller molecules of LDL that easily penetrate blood vessel walls, and cause a build-up of plaque, that interferes with blood flow.[22] He also suggests it is 'faulty thinking' that if you have plaque you're stuck with it, as he reckons his dietary ideas can reverse the process. More on this later.

Oxidative stress

Oxidation is what is happening when steel combines with oxygen and rusts. In the body, reactive unpaired oxygen atoms, called free radicals, damage proteins and genes in a process called oxidative stress. Basic functions including breathing and digestion cause this, as well as ultraviolet light, smoking, radiation, stress, pollution, a poor diet and infections. If a body has an excess of free radical damage going on, we say it is overwhelmed and may be associated with chronic diseases and accelerated ageing.

Free radicals are neutralised through relaxation and antioxidants like vitamins A, C and E, zinc, selenium, copper, manganese and co-enzyme Q10, found in many foods, especially those we call 'superfoods'.[23] An example of antioxidant action is lemon juice containing vitamin C, slowing the browning of a cut apple. Try naming some superfoods now and see how you fared when we get to the food chapter.

Chronic inflammation

Inflammation occurs when the body responds to incidents like injury and infection and is a key factor in many chronic (ongoing) diseases including asthma, rheumatoid arthritis, metabolic syndrome, multiple sclerosis and inflammatory bowel disease. One extensive study has also shown a link of the inflammatory process to heart disease, as measured by C-reactive protein.[24]

Dr D. Lundell, a heart surgeon with 25 years' experience, suggests inflammation is the real cause of heart and some chronic diseases. It seems the body's immune response cannot switch off, hence the expression 'autoimmune disease', where the body's immune system attacks body cells.

Why this happens is unclear and may be due to foreign materials that have entered the cells, poor diet, being overweight, ageing, physical inactivity, smoking, poor hygiene, stress, gingivitis (inflamed gums that might increase the risk of heart disease), high LDL-cholesterol and even certain bacteria in the colon that release antigens into the bloodstream to trigger an immune response.[25] Later we look at the anti-inflammatory effects of some fatty acids in food.

General stress

In today's complex world many experience stress, typically from over-reacting to stimuli. It can have serious consequences on mental and physical health, leading to unhealthy eating habits, lack of exercise, alcohol and drug abuse, anxiety, depression, poor immunity, cortisol overload, irritable bowel, lack of energy and heart disease. Researchers in Germany (Professor A. Zeiher) rate the consequences of stress as high as smoking and cholesterol problems, and highlight that even retirement can be a serious risk factor for some people.

Research even suggests stress triggers gene changes that threaten the health of future generations. Helping each other within a caring community is vital for health, with many opportunities to improve, including reducing the financial and emotional stress caused by the widening gap between house prices and incomes. We could also take a serious look at negative social influences such as crime and violence, we allow into our lives via the media and entertainment, and how we can reduce this; something I plan to cover in my next book.

De-stressing and relaxing is critical to good health, as shown by research. Using Magnetic Resonance Imaging (MRI), scans show that meditation can have a positive effect on the body and mind, including compassion, anxiety, substance abuse, chronic pain, depression, eating disorders, ageing, attention span, concentration, thinking and memory.

Many resources are available to help, including suggestions outlined by Goldie Hawn in *10 Mindful Minutes*, based on personal experience. She suggests we take time out to be self-aware, focus on the 'now,' not past woes, and be grateful for what we have, and combine this with hobbies and sports. Be careful about overdoing the relaxation though, as a recent meta-analysis review links more than three hours of television watching a day to Type 2 diabetes and heart disease.[26] [27]

How we live our lives can impact on our health, i.e. in Germany, a study involving 65,000 people over a 25 year period found those involved in actively helping people, or kept busy with family, were more satisfied and happier than those who focused on career success, and materialism. In the interests of your health, try focusing on as many positive, happy things as you can for 21 days or more, so they become a habit.

Start with a smile, mix with positive people, listen to lively music, laugh and be grateful for who you are and what you've got. If you have lost the zest for life, before you beat yourself up, consider medical causes like vitamin B deficiency or adrenal fatigue, where the adrenal gland has reduced production of key hormones like cortisol. Taking adaptogens, like ginseng, may help the body adapt to stress.

Research suggests 'planning your tomorrow' engages your brain to dream about it, which may help it happen and reduces stress. As you go to bed at night, consider analysing your day and program yourself for a great tomorrow. The '**B-Alert**' acronym from the book *The Power of Focus* is one way to do this, i.e. have a **b**lueprint (plan) for daily **a**ctivity; consider what you **l**earnt today, what **e**xercise and **r**elaxation you did, and what you **t**hink about your situation.[28]

Carry a 'grateful stone' in your pocket to remind you of how great life is, but remember happiness is not as easy to define as you might think. Some people confuse happiness with temporary incidents of feeling good through material things. Some experts suggest 50% of our happiness is in our genes; 35% how we think and 15% dependent on circumstances.

Considering the power of the mind and the impact of negativity on health, it is time we replaced broad terms like cancer (that covers a wide range of conditions and outcomes) with more focused terms to truly reflect prognosis etc.

We cannot be happy all the time, so it is okay to be sad.[29] When parents say 'I only want my children to be happy,' it is tempting to suggest how important it is for children to learn to cope with disappointment and unfairness in the world. Focusing on the positives is good, but so is being realistic.

Diabetes

We take a look at carbohydrates (carbs, sugars and starches) in the section on nutrition. For the time being, appreciate that insulin maintains ideal blood sugar (glucose) levels by balancing the absorption of glucose from the bloodstream into cells of your body for energy and the storage of excess as glycogen.

Diabetes is where this mechanism is out of balance. There is a limit to how much glycogen the body can store, so excess carbohydrates convert to triglycerides in the liver for storage as fat, also known as adipose tissue.[30]

Type 1 diabetes is an autoimmune disease that generally develops during childhood following destruction of the insulin-secreting beta cells of the

Islets of Langerhans in the pancreas, where insulin injections to are needed to control blood sugar levels. Type 2 diabetes is where: the body does not produce enough insulin, does not recognise that it is present, or where its effect is reduced (insulin resistance).

Diabetes is one of the fastest-growing diseases in the world. About 20 New Zealanders are diagnosed with it every day, with the cost of treatment expected to triple to $1.7 billion by 2021.[31] [32] In the USA, diabetes increased from 4% to 9% of the population in ten years (i.e. up to 2011.) An international study, published in the prestigious medical journal, *The Lancet* (June 2011) shows over 350 million people in the world have diabetes, a global health problem.

Some scientists blame the spread of the Western-style diet (discussed later) with rising levels of diabetes. It is the leading cause of heart and kidney disease, blindness, stroke and a lower limb amputation every thirty seconds, somewhere in the world.[33] Research is also linking the disease with dementia and memory loss.[34] [35] Drs Bruner and Rosser on the Dr Oz show made the claim that gastric bypass operations can reverse Type 2 diabetes quickly in morbidly obese patients.

Metabolic Syndrome (Syndrome X)

This disease is a cluster of conditions characterized by insulin resistance, Type 2 diabetes, high BP and dangerous visceral fat around the stomach and vital organs like the heart and kidney. One in three is likely to suffer from liver problems. About a fifth (20%) of our population has it, as do half (50%) of the obese.[36]

The condition is also associated with diseases like breast, prostate and colon cancer. Causes include poor diet, excess weight, genes, too little exercise, excessive alcohol, certain medicines, and possibly certain bacteria in the gut.[37]

Dental issues

Someone I know seriously damaged his teeth as a child by scrubbing across his teeth with too hard a toothbrush, exposing him to gingivitis, chronic inflammation, heart disease and stroke.

Brushing from the gums towards the teeth is ideal, yet we often see people brushing across their teeth in movies, etc. Food tends to make the mouth acidic, so you are more likely to damage tooth enamel if brush your teeth within an hour after eating.

Surveys have found about 35% of New Zealanders need dental treatment they're not getting, probably due to the relatively high cost. Some are opting to go overseas for cheaper treatment. Dr Mehmet Oz recommends digital dental X-rays whenever possible as they user lower levels of radiation. He also warns people to make sure dentists use a thyroid guard when doing an X-ray. (Find out more at www.doctoroz.com.)

Modern dentistry is steadily improving to make a visit more effective and less stressful.[38] Check with your dentist about improved technology available or consult websites like the New Zealand Institute of Minimal Intervention Dentistry (www.nzimid.org).

To complement visits to your dentist, consider using a battery operated, oscillating toothbrush that gives a better result than a manual brush, especially if it has a two-minute timer. For health teeth and gums, combine this with regular flossing and dental brushes that go between teeth to remove food, bacteria and plague.

With the controversy over people's rights, versus risk and benefit, one has to ask whether if it is better to focus on better lifestyles than fluoride, as most tooth decay is likely to be due to poor cleaning habits, fruit juice and soft drinks. Ideally, dilute juice with water, rinse the mouth with water after, or, better still, swap to whole fruits. Sadly, a survey of 1,000 people, done by drug company GlaxoSmithKline in 2012, found many respondents, who suffered from fruit juice damage to their teeth, said they were unlikely to change their habits.

Some experts urge caution on the use of alcoholic mouthwash due to a possible link to oral cancer. 'Alcohol free' products are now available.

Smoking

Many people die each year from smoking-related diseases, with one in two likely to die twenty years earlier than they should. Reducing the number of people smoking would significantly reduce health costs.

With this in mind, it is hard to fathom why a New Zealand-made television program (2011), on a state-owned enterprise channel, featured people smoking in a modern setting, when the government spends so much money trying to reduce the number of smokers through their quit program - Quitline (0800-778 778, www.quit.org.nz.)

Plans in New Zealand to stamp out smoking by 2025 include price hikes, disallowing advertising in shops and possibly forcing manufacturers to remove branding from their packs.

No doubt the companies will use all the tricks they can to remain in business, like those that encourage children in Africa to form the smoking habit, through sales of individual cigarettes, to reduce a price barrier.

CHAPTER 6

Germs and Immunity

Hygiene is a subject of immense breadth and depth. For our present purpose, which is to provide a broad overview, we will quickly run through some key points.

Micro-organisms (germs and microbes) include bacteria, parasites, viruses, algae and fungi; mostly invisible to the naked eye, meaning it is easy to forget they are swarming all around us. The weight of all micro-organisms on earth is 25 times that of all species of animals. The colon contains nine times as many bacteria as human cells in the body. Some are friends (probiotics) like 90% of the 1.5kg (100 trillion bacteria) in our gut. Some are foes that can cause serious disease and death.

Prions are infective particles easily transmitted via the blood or other bodily fluids. While most are harmless, some are responsible for previously unexplained conditions like mad cow disease (bovine spongiform encephalopathy, BSE.) An epidemic of this was caused when farmers, in their ignorance, fed cows bone meal that was contaminated with the prion.

In 2009, French officials were exonerated for authorising the use of growth hormone for children after it was later found to be contaminated with a variant of the prion affecting cows.

Bacteria multiply by splitting into two in a process called mitosis. Now consider that a single bacterium divides every thirty minutes. Assuming none die, how many descendants will it have in ten hours? Unbelievably, the answer is over one million, which should give you some idea why it is so important to keep unfriendly bacteria under control, especially as some, like *Salmonellae* that cause food poisoning, can live on surfaces for up to 24 hours.

Viruses are different in that they invade cells where they multiply, or lie dormant for years, waiting for the right time to strike. An example is the *Herpes simplex* type1 virus that can enter a baby's body through a kiss from an adult with a cold sore. Years later that virus, which has lain dormant, may erupt into a cold sore, usually when the person's immune system is in a weak state. Post-polio syndrome is another example of 'sleeping' viruses. Now we are seeing the serious effects of the Ebola virus.

Infections

The BBC documentary on the *History of Surgery* highlighted the fact that doctors initially would not accept the idea that micro-organisms caused infection.

To give you an idea of the effects of infections, let us examine a case in Auckland some years ago, where 84 people got Hepatitis A and one person died. The problem arose in an affluent suburb. Working backwards, an astute public health official linked the outbreak to contaminated blueberries from a North Island orchard. It seems a child with Hepatitis A was picking fruit on the orchard, with poor toilet facilities.

In another example, *Norovirus*, a common cause of diarrhoea, affects 50,000 New Zealanders each year. It is highly infectious and transferred via contaminated food or faeces. *Norovirus* has a rapid onset and recovery and can survive weeks in food, though cooking at an appropriate temperature kills it. Low humidity increases the spread. A vaccine is now being trialled.

Infections are more likely to spread when people are in close proximity or share facilities, e.g. a study from Otago University in New Zealand in 2011 found the incidence of infection inside hospitals (and as a cause of admission) is rising. In some cases infections spread via carriers, people who do not show symptoms, but transfer them to others through physical contact, droplet spread from coughs and sneezes or from sharing drinking glasses, etc.

Resistance and superbugs

Over the years we have seen the emergence of bacteria that have developed a resistance to antibiotics commonly used to treat infections. One that poses a serious risk is MRSA, i.e. methicillin (or multi-) resistant *Staphlococcus aureus* or 'golden staph.'

Since 2003, hundreds of soldiers involved in the Iraq and Afghanistan wars have developed infections arising from the bacteria *Acinetobacter baumannii*. This is so resistant to modern antibiotics that doctors have had to resort to using an older antibiotic with potentially serious side effects. It can survive on surfaces like cell phones for up to two weeks and is now widespread in many hospitals in the USA, according to the Centers for Disease Control and Prevention (CDC).

Another new superbug, first detected in 2013 is **CRE** (*carbapenem-resistant enterobacteriaceae*), sometimes referred to as 'the nightmare bacteria,' much feared by medical experts.

Resistance comes about mainly due to the inappropriate use of antibiotics, where bacteria get a chance to develop immunity to such treatments. This has prompted authorities to restrict the use of commonly used antibiotics like amoxycillin clavulanate to a narrow range of conditions. In addition, the European Union (EU) has banned the use of antibiotics as promoters of livestock growth. Use of antibiotics on the skin has also led to resistance and in most cases is closely controlled by regulation.

In Europe (2011) there was a major outbreak of food poisoning, caused by a strain of E coli, resistant to most treatments. This led to and incurred massive expenditure to investigate the source, treatment and destruction of vast amounts of contaminated bean sprouts.

In cases like this, expensive antibiotics are often required to treat resistant bacteria. However, because most antibiotic use is sporadic and short-term, there is no great incentive for drug companies to produce better ones. Concerns about the gravity of the situation have prompted professionals to urge governments to assist drug companies with research and development.

Some years ago, doctors were complaining of patient pressure to prescribe antibiotics, so the New Zealand Ministry of Health engaged in a program to educate the public that viruses are the cause of many winter infections, for which antibiotics are of no benefit. Patient pressure such as this can have serious consequences, as in one case where a doctor friend closed his practice in a rural town after false rumours spread that he was 'not much good,' because he refused to prescribe antibiotics that mothers (wrongly) believed their children needed. The message is clear that inappropriate use of antibiotics and bacterial resistant to them pose a very serious threat to world health, as outlined in a WHO report in 2014.

Toilet hygiene

By now you should have a greater appreciation of the importance of hygiene to health. Now let us consider some of the issues around toilet use, which can be a source of faecal-oral disease spread with virologists labelling diseases like polio as 'toilet diseases.'

At a seminar, it was discovered that unwrapped peppermints in a bowl had been contaminated with urine, through people not washing their hands. This led to the individual wrapping of such sweets, as seen today.

Consider toilet paper quality and thickness; don't economise with cheap brands. Use the hand least likely to touch food and consider how you can reduce contamination, e.g. by installing a bidet. Close the lid before flushing, to reduce contamination of the surrounding area, especially when toothbrushes etc. are in the same room.

Regarding hand washing, if possible, use an elbow to operate liquid soap dispensers and taps. In an ideal world, after washing hands, we should be able to exit toilets without the need to touch 'contaminated' doors, via a zigzag entrance, or a swing door you can push open without having to use your hands.

General hygiene

Keep your fingernails trimmed and clean. Wash and dry your hands thoroughly with soap and water for a minimum of 20 seconds (the time it takes to sing 'Happy Birthday'), or use alcoholic hand-rubs, especially after using the toilet and before eating or preparing food. Disposable paper towels and air dryers are preferred drying methods. This simple action can reduce sickness and time off school and work by 50%.

Infections can be spread by direct contact or aerosols (tiny droplets or particles suspended in air), that can travel a long way and stay aloft for a long time. To reduce this, cough or sneeze into your elbow to contain the spray in an area that is not likely to contaminate the air, others, or your hands. However, do not suppress coughing and sneezing, as this reduces your body's ability to eliminate allergens, microbes or toxins. Other key points are:

- Wear quality gloves and a mask when handling compost and potting mix, to avoid serious infections.
- Ensure wounds are appropriately covered.
- Hospitals are a 'meeting place' for infections where the need for correct hand washing is so serious some hospitals now use video cameras to monitor it.
- Wherever possible limit touching the hands of babies because they will likely transfer nasty bugs to their mouth.
- Germs may live on surfaces for days, so decontaminate kitchen benches, keyboards, phones, etc. regularly.
- Whenever possible, remove shoes when entering houses. The soles of your shoes may appear clean, yet provide a real opportunity to contaminate floors, especially carpets. Think twice about having wall-to-wall carpet, especially in food areas.
- Stay away from work, etc., if you have an infectious illness.
- Ventilation and adequate heating is important for health by reducing damp and mouldy conditions.
- Buy medicines in tubes rather than jars that are easily contaminated, if possible.

Food hygiene

To reduce food poisoning consider the following:

- Start with the Ministry of Health's '4Cs' i.e. <u>C</u>lean, <u>C</u>ook (to right temperature), <u>C</u>over and <u>C</u>hill. If you usually wear glasses, always do so to ensure adequate cleaning.

- Separate raw and cooked food and utensils, i.e. NEVER place cooked meat on the plate you used for the raw meat.

- Raw meat may contain harmful bacteria, so store it in a sealed container at the bottom of your refrigerator to reduce spread and wash your hands after handling.

- Foods like poultry, sausages and mince need to be thoroughly cooked with juices running clear and the meat a light grey colour. Ideally, for cooking or reheating, use a cooking thermometer to check internal temperatures. Figures vary from 60° to 90° C depending on the food. [www.foodauthority.nsw.gov.au]

- Keep hot food hot, cold food cold. Store left-over food in the fridge as soon as it stops steaming.

- Wear a clean apron when preparing food.

- Store all food in sealed containers to limit insect infestation and contamination.

- Wash produce in cold running water if you plan to eat it raw; otherwise, plate-up food using utensils, not hands.

- Avoid sharing food containers like glasses, cups and water bottles and do not place utensils you have had in your mouth in food other people will be eating.

- Always be on the lookout for potential contamination i.e. in *New Nutrition* by Michael Colgan cited instances of factory fish found to be contaminated with faecal bacteria, as a result of poor staff hygiene practices.[39]

- Check the temperature of your fridge regularly to ensure it is between 2-4°C and the freezer is below minus 18°C. Use a maximum-minimum thermometer in a clear container to give you time to note readings before they change.

- Use a dishwasher whenever possible. They rinse off detergent, are hygienic and economical with water, power and time. Avoid leaving dirty dishes that may grow bacteria in them for any lengthy periods.

- Keep dishcloths and tea towels as clean and dry as possible. Microwaving may help.

- Use separate cloths for 'clean' areas, e.g. a sink and 'dirty' areas, e.g. the floor.
- Beware of environments where you do not have control, i.e. restaurants. Check for evidence of certification, etc.
- Barbecues attract cockroaches, so clean the cooking surface well before use (i.e. water on a hotplate to steam clean it.)

The immune system

Your immune system comprises structures and processes that resist the attempts of environmental forces like infections, allergy and cancer to overrun, destroy or gain control of part of your body. It includes physiological barriers (body temperature and stomach acid); good bacteria (probiotics); various organs; cells and anatomic barriers (such as the skin, hair and mucous membranes).

Hair barriers like eyelashes protect your eyes from dust and debris. Mascara may counteracts this protection, so its use should be limited. On top of this, bacterial contamination of test bottles in stores that could cause infection have been seen.

When challenged by an invader, a complex cascade of actions involving macrophages, mast cells, phagocytes and white blood cells go into action to fight an infection.[40]

Paracetamol and non-steroidal anti-inflammatory medicines like ibuprofen, lower body temperature as well as relieving pain. With this in mind, a paediatrician in charge of a children's ward restricted their use because a moderate fever is part of the body's way of fighting infections, as some bacteria do not like higher temperatures. The key point is at what temperature do we intervene? Check out www.health.govt.nz for up to date information.[41]

Through the power of advertising, customers often came into our pharmacy to buy products to treat symptoms of colds and flu. Not only do some reduce fever, which, as we have seen, may not be ideal, some contained pseudoephedrine, which has adverse side effects and is not suitable to be used in some medical conditions. It was also being bought to make illicit methamphetamine (speed), so it is now a controlled drug in New Zealand and no longer used in over-the-counter (OTC) medicines.

While these 'cough and cold' products generally gave quick relief, we emphasised the importance of helping the body fight infections through a healthy immune system with immune-boosting products. These seemed to work well, as we often guaranteed them and not one person claimed their money back.

Products to boost immune cell response include vitamins A and C, zinc, selenium, colostrum, echinacea, astralagus, garlic, shitake mushrooms and olive leaf extract. In our pharmacy we often did a 'zinc taste test' to check body levels and found many people needed a boost, via food or supplements. It is interesting that medicines that unleash the power of the immune system on cancers are now generating considerable optimism.

Over ten years in our community pharmacy my wife and I took immune boosting supplements during the winter months. Even though we interacted with many infected patients, we did not get any significant infections. This does not absolutely prove the products worked, but again, absence of evidence is not evidence of absence.

The farming industry is currently experimenting with 'immune defence protein' in cows, with suggestions it may be trialled in humans.

An eye surgeon says he sees few infections when operating in parts of Asia in less than ideal conditions. This is likely because the people have strong immune systems through regular exposure to infections. In fact, some experts suggest we live in 'too sterile' an environment, including washing too much with alkaline soaps that irritate the skin and neutralise protective fatty acids. In fact, research demonstrated increased serotonin levels and happier rodents when they were infected with the bacteria *Mycobacterium vaccae*, indicating exposure to infections could have some added benefits.

Vaccines

The immune system takes time to develop antibodies to fight infections. While not all vaccinations work every time, they are a means of speeding up this process by exposing the immune system to non-infectious forms of bacteria, etc., so that the body is ready to fight, should the real infection appear. Some people, when exposed to serious infections, do not succumb, either because of previous mild exposure or because their immune system is strong enough to fight off the infection.

Hearing that a mercury preservative was added to some vaccines in the past alarms patients about safety issues. Information about side effects (that may be co-incidental and difficult to prove) is important to help them assess the risks and benefits and their responsibility to society.

With authorities working hard to increase the uptake of vaccination programs, it is unhelpful when a public health doctor says on television, "All the information about the risks with the vaccine would not fit on the official brochure." Neither is a statement from a nurse that she will not get a cold because she has had the flu vaccine.

Real transparency and knowledge is important to instil trust and public confidence, especially when recent research found the flu vaccine used in New Zealand at the time was 'only 50% effective.' Authorities tend to overlook issues including the importance of good hygiene and the power of fighting infections through a healthy immune system, and warning patients who may be more susceptible to infection because of the medicines they take, or diseases they have.

The documentary *Vaccine War* features a doctor who developed the Rotavirus vaccine in the USA saying, "It does not matter that I gain financially from sales of the product." Clearly, financial returns may affect ethics and honesty about safety, etc., especially when drug companies conduct most vaccine studies and fund some public health seminars.

Stomach (gut) bacteria

It seems undesirable changes in bacteria in our gastro-intestinal tract may be linked to diseases including Parkinson's, obesity, multiple sclerosis, Type 1 diabetes, chronic fatigue syndrome (CFS), rheumatoid arthritis and other autoimmune diseases.[42]

This idea evolved when doctors observed that some patients with a very serious gut infection, caused by the micro-organism *Clostridium difficile*, showed improvement in their Parkinson's disease when treated with a faecal (stool) transplant to recolonize the gut with good bacteria, lost through antibiotic use etc. This suggests it may be caused by a certain bacteria that enters the central nervous system.

We do not fully understand what constitutes 'healthy colon flora,' therefore large-scale faecal transplants from donors are unlikely at this stage, because of the risk of treating one disease and introducing another, but antibiotics may have a role.

Research also suggests there could be a link between obesity and microbes in your gut where certain bacteria cause release of nutrients in food that would have remained undigested in lean people.[43]

CHAPTER 7

Medicines and You

While some people use the words medicine and drug interchangeably, the Medicines Act and Regulations in New Zealand define a medicine as anything with a 'therapeutic' benefit. The term drug is reserved for 'drugs of abuse,' e.g. methamphetamine, as covered by the Misuse of Drugs Act.

Medicines go through four phases in the body, i.e. absorption; distribution to various parts of the body; breakdown by the body into forms that make it easier to excrete, and excretion. Medicines generally interact with receptors in the body, according to their molecular shape, akin to a key in a lock.

My guess is that 80% of today's medicines were not available in 1970 when I was training. With such a major and ongoing change, can you imagine the education required for doctors to keep up to date? Fortunately, most only use a small number in their everyday work.

Many medicines are derived from plants, with some altered to improve characteristics like duration of action, purity and potency. Also known as, pharmaceuticals, medicines have three names, as follows:

1. Chemical name - describes the structure of a molecule, usually used by scientists e.g. N-Acetyl-p-aminophenol.
2. Generic name - this is a user-friendly variation of the chemical name, e.g. paracetamol and acetaminophen (USA).
3. Brand (or trade) name – this is the unique name given to a company's product, e.g. Panadol.

Patents and generic medicines

Clearly to make a profit and stay in business, any drug company developing a new medicine needs to recoup more than the costs of research, development, production and marketing.

Currently the patent period for medicines in New Zealand is twenty years, with no extension allowable, as in some countries. It generally takes about fifteen years to achieve regulatory approval for distribution of a new medicine, so the time to recoup costs and make a profit is limited.

We use the term 'generic medicine' to describe medicines manufactured and supplied by companies after the original patent has expired. As they have not incurred the developmental and marketing costs of the original branded product, their prices are usually substantially lower. Manufacturers of original medicines may introduce a secondary brand as a patent expires, to reduce the impact of other generic medicines on the market.

Drug companies

Drug (pharmaceutical, medicine) companies have provided an extensive range of medicines to keep people alive and well, playing a significant role in how medicine has evolved. In the 1940s there were few medicines, but by the 1960s seventy new medicines a year were being introduced.

In 2003, the top medicines in the world were for cholesterol, schizophrenia, stomach problems, heart and blood pressure, asthma and anti-depressants, totalling over US$48 billion in turnover. Today in the USA the focus is on diabetes, rheumatoid arthritis, Alzheimer's disease, gene technology, and heart and airways disease.[44]

With the slowdown in new medicines, expiry of patents and a focus on generic medicines, drug company profitability has dropped, as reported in the *Harvard Business Review*. This probably explains why we are seeing more amalgamations, leading to a handful of 'Druggernauts.'

While there is the assumption that a higher price reflects more research, factors like marketing may account for as much as 36% of turnover. Much profit has been made out of successful medicines, with global spend increasing 25-fold over 25 years.

In some cases companies create business by raising attention to a particular condition, e.g. hormone replacement therapy for menopausal symptoms (now reduced due to side effects).

Drug companies may provide incentives for doctors to prescribe their products and compromise standards, so plans are underway in the USA to list relevant details on a website by 2015.

Side effects of medicines

Medicines provide benefits like reducing high blood pressure by relaxing the muscles of blood vessels so they dilate, or widen.

Medicines usually produce other (side) effects, some of which are useful, e.g. an antihistamine for allergic reactions that causes drowsiness may be good to sedate an agitated and very itchy patient. On the other hand, medicines may have negative (adverse) effects, as the following anecdote illustrates.

Not long after buying our community pharmacy, I met a patient taking an older medicine with a common adverse side effect of nightmares. I discovered he suffered from them and this caused him much distress. I started to tell him how we could fix the situation, but his wife quickly interrupted, stating that her husband's problem was none of my business. She added, "The doctor is the one looking after him."

A few days later, the man came back on his own asking for help. I rang his doctor and explained the situation. It turned out he had bought an older doctor's practice and was happy to change the prescription to a modern medicine that was less likely to cause the adverse effect. The nightmares stopped and the patient was delighted. This was one of many cases where I was able to improve things.

In another incident, a patient came into our pharmacy to buy some cough mixture. I suggested the 'ACE inhibitor' medicine he was taking was the likely cause of his cough and asked if I could discuss this with his doctor. He declined, probably because he did not want to create a fuss, a situation we often encountered, especially with older patients. After he left the pharmacy, I decided to act in his best interest, and rang his doctor's surgery. As the doctor was not available, I explained the situation to the nurse. Unbelievably she told me, "Mind your own business. The doctor is in charge."

My response was that medical ethics require professionals like her to do things like watching for common side effects such as their patient was experiencing. I tell this story not to denigrate professionals, as most are doing a good job, but to impress upon you that professionals do not always work in your best interest.

Medicines play a key role in keeping us alive. However, we must treat them with caution, as a number have been subsequently withdrawn due to adverse effects, even death. Some medicines like thalidomide attracted widespread attention because of drastic and unanticipated side effects, whereas others were quietly withdrawn and drug companies have paid out large sums of money in fraud cases. Clearly the more people are aware of issues surrounding their medicine treatment, the greater the chances of reducing the risks.

Elderly patients take most medicines, yet few studies involve this age group. As a result, side effects relevant to older patients may emerge much later, emphasising how important it is to report any unexpected effects, no matter how insignificant they seem to be. Side effects may take years to emerge, as in the case of girls developing cancer whose mothers had taken a hormonal medicine before their birth.

As we increase the dosage of a medicine, typically benefits tail off and side effects increase. The trick is to get the balance between a dose that is working and a dose where side effects become a problem. In blood pressure control, it is easy to see if a medicine is working, but not so easy in conditions like depression.

A side effect rated common is when one in 100 people experience it and uncommon if one in a 1,000 or more experience it. Some patients do not notice side effects, especially if the onset is slow. Others put them down to 'old age' and for some they can be serious enough to need a change of medicine.

"What did your doctor tell you about your medicine?" was my standard question when dispensing prescriptions for new medicines. In too many cases, the answer was, "Nothing," although in some cases I think they had just forgotten.

This emphasises the need for written material and for health professionals to ensure proper understanding of medicines and how to use them. I have even known doctors who did not want patients to know anything about possible side effects of medicines taken because they believed 'they will imagine they've got them and stop taking their medicine.' Now that most patients have ready access to the Internet etc., this approach is futile and misses an opportunity to tailor information to patients.

Polypharmacy

About 40% of the New Zealand population are taking at least one medicine by age 60 with numbers increasing dramatically by age 75. Polypharmacy describes situations where a patient takes around five or more medicines.

Typically this occurs when a condition like high blood pressure may require a number of medicines, each acting differently to achieve control. In other examples, patients have a number of diseases, involving a variety of specialists.

An example of challenges that can arise from such a situation occurred years ago, when a new eye drop, prescribed by eye specialists for glaucoma, led to some patients developing asthma, the cause of which sometimes took time to resolve.

I once worked with two hospital doctors who specialised in treating elderly patients. The doctors felt too many patients were coming into hospital on more medicines than necessary and worked hard to rationalise treatment. However, I saw cases where local doctors rejected such changes and put patients back onto their own treatment, after discharge.

In one instance a local doctor stopped a cholesterol medicine prescribed by a hospital heart specialist for a patient admitted after a heart attack. When I questioned why it was missing from her next prescription, the doctor said, "The high cost could not be justified at her age." I rang the specialist and suggested he discuss the matter with the woman's doctor. Sadly, he was not prepared to do so and shrugged off the issue, saying, "The local doctor is in charge of the patient."

I wonder what the patient, her family and administrators would have said, had they known about this, especially as this story played out again after a subsequent heart attack.

Medicine interactions

I recall the case of a woman admitted to hospital in a serious condition after taking some of her husband's anti-depressant medicine prescribed for sleep. This resulted in a serious interaction with a different anti-depressant she was taking. Interactions like this can occur in the body between medicines, supplements, herbs and food, e.g. antibiotics may kill vitamin K-producing bacteria in the stomach, increasing the effect of some medicines that slow clot formation.[45]

Some antibiotics kill good acidophilus bacteria (probiotics) in the stomach, upsetting the balance, which may lead to thrush or diarrhoea. To counter this, a dose of billions of acidophilus bacteria (often not achievable with commercial yoghurt) taken in capsules may help. Especially if taken at least two hours away from the antibiotic, (to reduce the chances of it killing the good bacteria) or after the course. If travelling, consider this treatment to reduce your chances of contracting traveller's diarrhoea, especially with brands that can be stored at room temperature.

Food interactions are many including tea, coffee and some spices that deplete zinc and reduce iron absorption, if taken at the same time.[46]

There is a growing awareness of the importance of reporting unexpected effects, which may lead to the discovery of a new interaction that others have ignored or not reported. This can be significant as interactions may take some time to identify and prove, as in the discovery that eating grapefruit could adversely affect how some medicines work.

Proving an interaction when the patient takes two medicines is relatively straightforward, but gets complicated if they're on a cocktail of medicines. On top of this, the body usually metabolises medicines into other chemicals to facilitate excretion, increasing the potential for further interactions.

A news story in New Zealand some years ago reported the deaths of two people from the effects of statin medicines, taken to control cholesterol. The nub of the story was that the deaths might have been prevented, had they reported symptoms of a serious problem called rhabdomyolysis (muscle pain, tenderness or weakness), linked to reduced levels of coenzyme Q10 (CoQ10) in the body. While few patients with these symptoms are likely to have rhabdomyolysis, it still needs investigating.

Older people, especially those taking statin medicines may benefit from foods that contain CoQ10, including chicken, sardines, mackerel, nuts and some organ meats, or as a supplement taken with some fat to help absorption. Health benefits include improved circulation, increased energy and a potent antioxidant activity (discussed later.) [47] [48] Sometimes the reduced form, ubiquinol, is recommended over the original ubiquinone. However, David Coory, author of the invaluable guide *Stay Healthy by Supplying What's Lacking in your Diet* says, "This is not necessary, unless doses over 200mg per day are needed. Ubiquinol is more expensive and has a shorter shelf life." [49]

This interaction has been so hotly debated Dr J. M. Whitaker sued the FDA for refusing to change the warning labels on statin medicines to inform healthcare practitioners and consumers that the medicines deplete coenzyme CoQ10 levels. The FDA admit that statins lower CoQ10, but refused to put consumers on notice, holding the view that the evidence of harm was not strong enough to warrant this. As a precaution, our pharmacy labelled statin medicines with 'Report any muscle pain, tenderness of weakness immediately to your doctor.'

Soon after the television report on the deaths of the two patients mentioned above, I rang the Centre for Adverse Reactions to Medicines (CARM) in Dunedin New Zealand and suggested they put out a public warning about the problem. They said it was not their role and told me to ring the Ministry of Health, where I spoke to a doctor who surprised me by saying, "We don't have a way to communicate with the public of New Zealand."

To improve awareness of interactions between medicines, food and supplements, Blackmore's, a supplier of vitamin and mineral supplements, introduced a computer software system in 2011, to suggest diet considerations for use by pharmacists, when dispensing prescriptions. An influential doctor interviewed on Radio New Zealand National about the project dismissed it, saying, "It is just a ploy to increase sales."

Such narrow-mindedness tells us there is still some way to go before we achieve a transparent and wholistic 'big picture' approach to health, especially as the software might have prevented those two deaths, mentioned earlier.

Blackmores have dropped the project for now, due to the negative reaction. In time, I am sure, software like this will become widespread, providing important information, even for patients not taking medicines, but who have conditions linked to nutritional factors, discussed later.

Wise use of medicines

By now I trust you have a good overview of key issues surrounding the proper use of medicines. We will look at some practical issues surrounding medicine prescriptions in the pharmacist section. For now, consider the following.

A paramedic told me he sees patients using their angina spray for coughs and colds, leading to complications because it drops their blood pressure. This is a reminder for patients to know; what their medicine is for, side effects, precautions, when to take, what to do if a dose is missed and interactions with alcohol, other medicines, supplements and food. Follow instructions carefully. If you are not sure what to do, do not be afraid to ask, as the only dumb question is the question unasked.

A teenage boy nearly shared his acne medicine with his girlfriend. As it causes significant birth defects, this could have had disastrous consequences. Because he was a male, it is likely this side effect was not emphasised. The moral of the story, NEVER share prescription medicines with others.

Know if it is safe to drive or operate machinery while taking a particular medicine. Under the Drug Driving program, New Zealand police can now check for medicines affecting driving, i.e. opiates, amphetamines, antidepressants, cannabis, sedatives and methadone.[50] However, the program does not include medicines that cause problems like blurred vision and light-headedness. How long a medicine works in the body is variable, so while you might not feel sleepy, a medicine you took last night may make you unsafe today, slowing your reflexes or affecting your ability to concentrate on demanding tasks like driving or operating machinery. Other key points include:

- Always tell health professionals what medicines and supplements you're on; ideally, take them along to your consultations. Realise they might not know about some supplements, so you may need to provide details for them.

- Most medicines simply control symptoms of diseases so need to be taken regularly to work.

- Chronic (ongoing) pain medicines work better if taken regularly to keep pain under control.

- Complete courses of antibiotics to reduce resistance, unless prevented by side effects.

- Most medicines taken orally are better absorbed if downed with a glass of water.

- Keep all medicines out reach of children. Medicines like morphine are of interest to drug users, so keep them out of sight. Even a casual comment by a visitor to someone in the community could set you up for a robbery.

- Ask if sugar-free syrups are available, to reduce tooth decay.

- Return unused medicines to your pharmacy for appropriate disposal, to avoid environmental pollution caused if they are flushed down drains, toilets, etc.
- Check if a medicine contains ingredients you need to avoid e.g. gluten.
- Liquids in a measure have a curved meniscus on the surface, caused by liquid creeping up the sides. Read measurements from the bottom of this curve.[51]
- Certain medicines are illegal in some sports.
- Avoid aspirin in children, unless advised otherwise by a health professional.

CHAPTER 8

Health Professionals

Following claims of an unethical experiment at National Women's Hospital in the late 1980s, an inquiry by Judge Dame Sylvia Cartwright followed with the enactment of the Health and Disability Act, with a clear objective of protecting patients from inappropriate medical behaviour by making professionals more accountable for their actions.

Most health professionals do a great job. However, as I've worked alongside hundreds, it would be negligent of me to simply paint a rosy picture, and ignore the fact they're human and may make mistakes. Most learn from those mistakes and are the better for it. The following stories give some idea of issues.

During my training a lecturer taught pharmacology (medicine action) from a textbook and had little 'real world' clinical input. After graduating I went on a course conducted by a medical specialist, who not only treated hospital and private patients, but also had a degree in pharmacology. The difference in the quality of information and learning was huge, because he was able to relate theoretical knowledge to real and unique patients taking medicines, with real diseases and laboratory results etc.

There was a time when I was teaching nurses about medicines, and discovered they memorised formulae to do dosage calculations. I saw the mistakes they made doing it like that and advised them to switch to a safer and more logical 'simple proportion' method.

An inquiry (2012) into midwifery mishaps in New Zealand recommended linking new graduates to mentors they've never been involved with to reduce compromised standards through friendships etc.

A health professionals' conference in New Zealand (2011), found their physical, emotional or mental condition adversely affected the ability of some attendees to do their jobs, with some being monitored to assess if they were fit to continue working. It recognised a need for more emphasis on self-care in training.

In the section on perception, we saw the work done by plastic surgeon Dr M. Maltz. In the introduction to his book, he says he was originally reluctant to publish his psychological findings because he felt his psychiatric colleagues would not approve of him writing about psychiatry when he was a plastic surgeon. Hopefully this sort of attitude has disappeared.

In 2011, a documentary featured US soldiers who had amputations during wars. One soldier displayed an expensive, computer-controlled artificial leg that allowed him to snowboard and lead a normal life. He now mentors soldiers with disabilities and runs seminars in armed services and civilian hospitals, highlighting how lives can be severely limited because of the attitudes of some health professionals. Instead of inspiring people to achieve great things like his snowboarding, he says they were often unaware of what was available, or had limited expectations of outcomes, resulting in 'less than satisfactory' service.

These examples (combined with the fact that rarely do exams test everything in a course) demonstrate that qualifications do not guarantee how well people perform at work. Ironically, some patients judge the competency of their health provider by 'how nice they are.'

Barriers to communication

Let us look at a few examples to see how easily communication can fail or compromise outcomes, e.g. many professionals use the term 'blood thinners' to describe medicines that slow the blood's clotting process. I recently heard a haematologist (blood specialist) use the term at a conference and raised the point that the emotive description might scare patients off taking their medicine. He agreed with me, and pledged not to use the term again.

Imagine a pharmacist has dispensed a prescription for an antibiotic for you. The label says 'Take one capsule four times a day on an empty stomach.' How would you interpret this? Would you take all doses by lunchtime or spread them throughout a 24-hour period? What do you understand by the term empty stomach? The stomach is empty just before a meal, but the intention here is that the medicine is swallowed one hour before or two hours after food, as some medicines are then better absorbed.

In another example, a doctor asks a patient if his pain is chronic. Thinking 'chronic' meant 'really bad' he answers 'no.' The point is that some health professionals use the term chronic to describe ongoing conditions, so the doctor got the wrong information, as the patient's pain was present all the time.

Type 2 diabetes was previously called 'mature-onset diabetes' because it mainly occurred in older adults. Today we see teenagers with the condition. Had we retained the original descriptive terminology, I believe more people would have asked why the condition was affecting younger people, which would have attracted attention to causes like insulin resistance much sooner than actually happened.

At a conference a skin specialist, newly arrived from overseas, said she tells patients to ignore how authorities in New Zealand tell pharmacists to label anti-inflammatory steroid creams, e.g. 'Apply sparingly,' as she wants the cream to be used liberally in some conditions. I suggested she talk to authorities and explain her point of view. In my experience, most people will not do this, probably because they see the process as being too hard, or fear repercussions.

Body language is an important part of communication as it gives clues to what a person is thinking.[52] For some patients, even a desk between them and their professional may affect their ability to feel comfortable enough to discuss key aspects of their health.

I trust the above examples give you a feel for the consequences of communication breakdown in health. Because patients come from different backgrounds and with different levels of education, it is important for health professionals to avoid medical jargon (terminology unique to a profession, group or event) that is likely to be unintelligible to patients.

Health professionals should heed what George Bernard Shaw once said. "The single biggest problem in communication is the illusion that it has taken place."

Reflective listening, where a patient repeats what they have been told, is one means of defeating such illusions. The acronym '**assume**' emphasises what happens otherwise, i.e. it makes an **ass** out of yo**u** and **me**.

Have you noticed how someone will say they agree with you, then negate it by adding 'but' and put forward their own idea? In this situation, motivational speaker Anthony Robbins suggests we listen respectfully to another's point of view, and then respond with 'That's interesting' and comment, if necessary.[53] Positive listening like this means focusing on what's being said, not detracting from it by thinking about what your response will be and interrupting before they have finished.

Consultations with health professionals

Research done by the Reverend Dr Robert Bayley of Los Angeles demonstrates how perception affects relationships with health professionals. He stresses the importance for health providers to ask probing questions like "Do you want to get well?" to unearth negative beliefs that could affect treatment outcomes where the patient might feel they're too old, or 'paying for their sins' or have given up hope.

Naturally it works both ways, so a health practitioner's worldview may affect outcomes, e.g. Dr Cantu, Professor of Neurosurgery in Boston, USA, says, "Females generally have weaker muscles, and their brains are not as well-protected as male brains, so they are more susceptible to concussion. Ignorance of this causes some male doctors to treat females with concussion less seriously than they should.'[54] This is particularly important, as head injury has links to dementia, Parkinson's disease and permanent brain damage.

Other examples of perception affecting professional-patient relationships include beliefs that a particular disease is a crutch for malingerers and patients who are well-informed about their condition can be difficult to treat, when others would say the opposite is true.

Dr Andrew Weill MD, wholistic health guru and founder of the Arizona Centre for Integrative Medicine, in the USA says, "Your doctor (and other health providers) should be a model of health, showing, rather than just telling you how to live a healthy life." Bear this valuable lesson in mind when assessing professionals to take care of your most valuable asset: your health. In some countries, there are websites where the public can rate health providers.

Some patients are negative about professionals who look up information. My advice is to have confidence in someone prepared to confirm facts, rather than rely on memory. I have also heard patients say. "My doctor thinks more about the computer than me," not appreciating that the doctor is simply using a tool to provide good treatment and keep records up to date.

In our pharmacy, we focused on being approachable and complemented this with a private counselling area, where patients often told us important things they had not mentioned to their doctor, so we did. The common reason given was 'I didn't want to trouble doctor.' We found this situation incredibly ironic as they paid the doctor to look after them (and so did the government) yet overlooked unpaid time we gave them.

Now let's consider how to prepare for a consultation. Some doctors get patients to complete a detailed questionnaire and send it to them before a consultation so it can be inputted into computer systems. Not only does this facilitate the process, it jogs the memory about symptoms that could be a clue to serious disease.

Close to the visit, consider phoning to check they are running on time, especially if you must travel a long distance. I once travelled for over an hour to find I had a three-hour wait, and was tempted to send the surgeon an account for time off work.

It is a good idea to take along a detailed record of events, as your memory may not be as reliable as you think. Jot down any questions you want to ask. Take along any prescription medicines, supplements and over the counter (OTC) medicines you're using. Taking along a support person is also a good idea; two heads are better than one to listen, remember details and discuss matters afterwards.

Some people have to take time off work to visit health practitioners, so extended hours are helpful, especially for those reluctant to go to after-hour practices.[55] Ensure you have adequate time to deal with all your issues. Some doctors require patients to book longer sessions if they wish to raise more than a couple of issues, which is worthwhile to ensure your doctor deals with the 'big picture.'

Along these lines, a doctor I know suggests he needs about half an hour with most patients to do the job thoroughly. When you consider the amount the patient and the government subsidy pays, maybe he should only see two patients per hour to legitimately call himself professional.

Do not be afraid to get involved in your treatment by asking why they are doing certain things, and beware of doctors terminating your visit too early, by reaching for a prescription pad. If you forget to ask something or do not understand something during a consultation, a quick phone call or email may resolve this without need for another consultation. If communicating this way, ensure accountability by knowing the staff member's name.

Written information

A Public Health Organisation (PHO) official had concerns that local/family doctor messages were not getting through to patients. This is not surprising when you consider the barriers to communication, combined with the fact that typically, patients receive a lot of verbal information in a relatively short visit with health professionals.

In light of this, just as public hospitals give patients a copy of discharge letters they send to family doctors, modern technology provides an opportunity for doctors to print details of diagnosis, treatment, laboratory results, etc., for patients to take away. This makes it easier for them to discuss issues with others.

Personal health records

There was a time when authorities had a plan for all patients to carry a 'smart card' with their medical history on it, but that idea appears to have slipped into oblivion.

Some people think all records on computers in the New Zealand health sector are connected, which is not the case. However, websites like www.managemyhealth.co.nz and www.health365.co.nz have emerged, where professionals send details of allergies, medical treatment, tests, etc., so patients can access the information. Of course, a simple folder may be a suitable alternative for some.

Not only does this tool involve patients in their own care, it gives them the ability to share and discuss their health information with family and friends - and patients can allow health professionals to access the information via the Internet when on holiday etc. It also enables health professionals to work collaboratively to provide safe, effective, and cost effective care. However, some professionals may be reluctant to adopt the systems, out of a fear of repercussions from mistakes etc.

A second opinion

A urinary tract surgeon (urologist) saw a two-year old child and wanted to do tests requiring a general anaesthetic. Unsure what to do, the parents consulted another urologist, who said the problem would disappear in a few months, which happened. Consider the anxiety of the parents had they taken the advice of the first specialist, after release of a retrospective study of 5,000 children who had had a general anaesthetic, which found an increase in learning disorders, especially with two or more exposures.[56]

In another example, a girl went to an orthodontist who planned to brace her teeth to straighten them. Friends recommended another opinion, resulting in extraction of a tooth on each side of the mouth at a fraction of the cost and all is well 25 years later.

Then there is the case involving a friend who asked his dental surgery (No.1) for information on flossing. They had none yet did not offer to get something for him even though he had just paid $300 for a filling. Frustrated, he changed to dentist No.2, where he was told the filling done by dentist No.1 was inappropriate because it would not stand up to the pressure of his tight jaw clench and would only last five years which turned out to be true.

Confused by opposing views, he saw an ad for a free check-up and decided to get another opinion (No.3), where he received a recommendation to have all his mercury amalgams replaced with modern fillings, at a cost of $11,000, with only a 5-year guarantee. The patient took digital X-rays from dentist No.3 back to dentist No.2 who said they were inadequate and needed repeating.

Dentist No.4 had doubts about the safety and reliability of modern fillings and described the quote as 'ridiculous and entrepreneurial.' Getting a second opinion can certainly add to the confusion. However, with more people choosing that option we are likely to see improvements in service and more competitive prices.

In some cases the outcome can be life-changing, like the girl with cerebral palsy whose parents did not accept the poor prognosis given by local doctors. Instead they took her overseas to consult a surgeon who dramatically improved her condition.

Some patients get agitated when their regular health professional is not available and they have to see someone else. What they do not appreciate is that sometimes it's good to have their situation reviewed by someone else, with a different worldview and knowledge base. In our pharmacy, we noted times when locum (relieving) doctors improved treatment, likely following a thorough examination of patients new to them.

Even doctors get second opinions when they present patients to colleagues for discussion, and sometimes two experts read medical scans to reduce errors. In fact, an Italian study found some melanoma surgeries done around the world were unnecessary, something that might not have occurred had doctors, or patients, sought a second opinion.

Medical decisions are generally not clear-cut, and as we only have one body, it is important to have a good quality assurance system, which might include a second opinion. It is not about a lack of confidence or trust, but of ensuring the best of care. Remember health professionals are human and this means they can have a bad day; a second opinion ensures you don't become a victim of that day. It also sends a clear message to professionals that they need to provide the best care possible to stay in business.

In the final analysis, it is vitally important to have a good health provider you can relate to and trust. If not, you have the option to try others, and when you find someone suitable, you can authorise them to transfer your medical records, so you don't have to do it. Check to ensure there is continuity of government subsidies with your change, as there was a time when paperwork took up to three months.

Waiting lists

One day a patient limped into our pharmacy with a prescription for painkiller medicines. His doctor had told him he would have to wait nine months for hernia surgery in a public hospital, as he could not afford private care. I asked if he thought he was getting a fair deal, to which he responded with a very definite "No!" I referred him to a Health Consumer Services mediator, resulting in his operation being done in a public hospital soon after.

Given how quickly this happened, I wonder why his doctor had not done what I did. Maybe he did not know the mediator service existed, or he was simply not prepared to advocate more strongly for his patient.

Some years ago, I asked an orthopaedic (bone) surgeon whether his waiting list (that stretched for months) concerned him. He casually replied, "For me a waiting list is part of my job and will always be there."

If you are on a waiting list, keep a close watch on your status to ensure you remain on it and are not downgraded, like the time when authorities shortened lists, by changing the criteria and dropping off patients. Some patients are stoic and reluctant to draw attention to their plight out of a belief that it is not right to jump the queue, when, in reality, it is about priority and fairness, as in the case of a friend, who waited patiently for six months for a scan.

I suggested he follow this up and interestingly his scan happened two days later. Unfortunately, they found a problem and one wonders how different his situation might be have been had the scan been done in a more timely manner. Sometimes it is all about the squeaky wheel getting the oil.

CHAPTER 9

Complementary Medicine

In our pharmacy, we did not promote the orthodox treatment for cold sores, simply because we felt it was relatively expensive and people had to apply it every four hours, while awake. In addition, the evidence at the time suggested the treatment would only reduce the duration by two to three days. We promoted foods, tablets and lip balms containing the amino acid, lysine and got fabulous results correcting a deficiency to improve their immune system's ability to deal with the infection.

Interestingly, the lip balm is no longer available, probably because of a false belief that the heavily-marketed medicines (with lower prices following the expiry of patents) are the best option.

Some years ago, a fascinating read was *The Liver Cleansing Diet* by Dr Sandra Cabot, a medical specialist from Australia, who found many of her patients had problems that she associated with liver toxicity. She developed methods to cleanse and detoxify this very important organ, including healthy raw food smoothies.[57] [58] She was a true pioneer, prepared to venture outside her original orthodox training to find answers, including smoothie recipes for different medical conditions.

Along these lines, patients suffering from gallstones might also find *The Amazing Liver and Gallbladder Flush* by Andreas Moritz helpful.[59]

Complementary and alternative medicine (CAM) includes acupuncture, aromatherapy, Ayurveda, chelation, chiropractic, colon cleansing, dark field microscopy, digital pulse analysing, fasting, herbs and spices, homeopathy, hyperbaric oxygen, hypnotherapy, iridology, kinesiology, liver detoxification, magnetic therapy, manipulative therapy, massage, meditation, nutrition, thermography, yoga and a variety of supplements. Some are simply part of everyday life, e.g. cycling may be helpful for Parkinson's disease and animals can warn of impending medical crises like heart and low blood sugar (hypoglycaemic) attacks.

Most holistic naturopaths (CAM practitioners) adhere to the six principles of naturopathy, i.e. promote the healing power of nature; prevention is the best cure; do no harm; treat the whole person and the cause, and the practitioner is the teacher. They aim to bring about balance to the body, using a variety of disciplines that arose from the Hippocratic School of Medicine in about 400 B.C.

Natural supplements are big business today, with a wide range available, including fish oil, glucosamine, grape seed extract, ginkgo biloba, saw palmetto, St. John's Wort, echinacea, melatonin, cinnamon, arginine, garlic, hawthorn, cayenne, manuka-honey dressings, capsaicin ointment, ginger and black cohosh. Consult with appropriately qualified health practitioners to guide you.

Quality standards

Some CAM products and practices are substantiated by research, e.g. a study in the USA (2009) involving 600 people with back pain showed a 40% improvement with conventional treatment increased to 60% when combined with acupuncture. For some, 'evidence' is use over centuries, without adverse effects.

Conventional research methods may not always apply because the mode of action of some natural products is different to medicines, and science tends to dislike models that do not fit with established theories. Where belief is part of treatment, results could be erroneous if patients know they might be taking a placebo.

Dr Ben Goldacre suggests some complementary practitioners lack self-appraisal and acceptance that the placebo effect may explain why some products and procedures work, as is the case for some medicines.[60]

While some supplements are ideal, others do not meet quality standards, e.g. some weight-loss products had to be withdrawn from the market in the USA, because they contained a prescription medicine. Be on the lookout for dodgy products and avoid those marketed in a foreign language, with no company name and address or that make unrealistic claims.

Sorting the wheat from the chaff can be difficult, but most would agree with *Consumer* magazine in New Zealand that 'dietary supplements need to be regulated, to ensure consumers are getting high-quality products that meet their claims.'

However, there was an emotional response and public opposition when the government of the time considered adopting an agreement with Australia to do that. The feeling was that the regulations went too far, restricting people's rights to access natural products.

The idea was canned but there are plans for a Natural Health Products Bill with the regulator, a unit (advised by a technical expert advisory committee) within the Ministry of Health, but separate from the medicines regulator, Medsafe.[61]

Patents

As discussed in the medicine section, legislation provides new medicines with a patent period, providing time for companies to reap the rewards of their research, development, production, marketing and sales. However, patent protection does not apply to natural products like vitamins and minerals, which limits prospects for good research.

To give you some idea of the issues, consider the 2011 story of a man who requested high dose injections of vitamin C for his swine flu and leukaemia. When staff at Auckland Hospital refused to give the injection, a senior doctor, interviewed on television said, "There was no research to prove its effectiveness." When asked, "Who will pay for the research on this natural nutrient without a patent?" he suggested it was up to those pushing the idea. Some doctors are encouraged by results with this treatment. [www.healthfreedom.co.nz]

Garlic, used in cooking for centuries, is considered to help conditions like adverse cholesterol levels, high blood pressure and infections. Let us say you decide to produce a garlic tablet and invest $1 million in researching its benefits. Can you see how your competitors will have the financial advantage, using the results of your research to promote their own sales? To get around this, some companies patent product-manufacturing processes.

The disease eclampsia can cause convulsions and raise blood pressure in pregnancy. It causes 50,000 deaths per year, mostly in the developing world. As far back as 1907, professionals had an idea that cheap, un-patentable magnesium would help, but it took until 2002 for the United Nations to recognise it as the 'best treatment.' This is an example where governments may have to step in and do research that private enterprise is unwilling to do, because, no patent means no exclusivity and no profitability.

Changing attitudes

In 1999 *The Arthritis Cure* by Dr Jason Theodosakis promoted the benefits of glucosamine and chondroitin in osteoarthritis.[62] Finding the concept of interest, I discussed it with colleagues.

Some showed a cynicism that had me wondering why intelligent professionals were not prepared to open their minds to new ideas. It is noteworthy that the authors highlighted the hazards of some non-steroidal anti-inflammatory medicines (NSAIDs), which proved to be correct, as some have been withdrawn from the market because of serious side effects, even death.

Interestingly, an orthopaedic surgeon told me in 2012 he thinks glucosamine and chondroitin is helpful for some patients, just as some medicines work in some people, and not others.

Some years ago I suffered a bout of vertigo (dizziness.) A medical specialist diagnosed BPPV (benign paroxysmal positional vertigo) and said all he could offer me were medicines. He then recalled that a surgeon had sent him an article about a new procedure called 'Canalith-repositioning exercises.' Although he did not think much of the 'alternative' idea, I was desperate for answers and implored him to try it, and it worked.

Ironically, the specialist did not follow me up, to see if it had worked, and this relatively simple procedure is now standard treatment for the condition. Go to www.youtube.com and search for 'Epley manoeuvre' and 'Brandt-Daroff exercise for BPPV' for more information.

Many people use some form of complementary therapy, yet most orthodox health professionals receive little, if any, training in these disciplines. Many rate their knowledge as inadequate and are not confident answering patient enquiries about this. However, we are seeing greater acceptance of complementary therapies, with some doctors undertaking training in some disciplines. Others are working collaboratively with CAM practitioners.

A place to start is with *Natural Remedies That Really Work* by Dr S. Holt, an orthodox doctor who came to appreciate the benefits of some natural healing, following his research.[63]

A key issue is that orthodox practitioners are likely to do alternative therapies in the same manner in which they practise orthodox medicine, which may set them up for failure.

With increased interaction between professionals, we will likely see less tunnel vision, more research and acceptance of other disciplines, rather than suspicion and derogatory comments that confuse and upset patients. For example, during one of my seminars, a chiropractor called out, "Doctors are poisoning patients with what they call medicines."

Unprofessional behaviour like this can do serious damage, undermining people's confidence in a health system that does much good work, even though there is room for improvement. A key for the future is to have more professionals appreciate the merits of a wholistic 'big picture' approach.

This reminds me of the farce some years ago, when there was a medical outcry to restrict royal jelly, following a death due to an allergic reaction to it, yet adverse effects of medicines often fly under the radar, and not all medicine is evidence-based.[64] When you consider that a number of medicines have been withdrawn because of adverse effects, including death, quality natural supplements are relatively safe.

That said, it is ideal to use complementary treatments in conjunction with appropriately qualified health practitioners, especially if you are on orthodox treatment. Do not be like some patients who replace medicines with natural supplements, without telling their orthodox health professionals, because they perceive 'Natural as better,' which is not always true, as previously discussed.

CHAPTER 10

Improving Medicine Use

Not to take anything away from other health professionals, I guess being a qualified pharmacist for over forty years qualifies me to give you some insight into pharmacy, and ways improve medicine use.

To qualify requires five years of tertiary training in a myriad of subjects including psychology, statistics, physiology, chemistry, biology, health, business management, hygiene and medicines. The course includes a final year, working under the supervision of a mentor pharmacist. Specialist areas include education, research, industry, hospitals, clinical and community pharmacy.

Following the Cartwright inquiry and legislation that followed, the responsibility of professionals like pharmacists is clear, to use their knowledge to ensure quality of care, i.e. they are accountable for correcting prescription errors, etc., and for acting in the best interests of patients, not just following doctors' orders on prescriptions, as some think.

How your pharmacist can help you

When I left Tauranga Hospital, my wife and I bought our community pharmacy. One of the first things we did was to put up a sign that advised: 'Please ensure you allow the pharmacist adequate time to give your prescription the due care and diligence it deserves.'

We did this because we found people did not value what we did for them. They tended to judge us by our speed in dispensing prescriptions, and availability of 'free' advice.

Much of the work pharmacists do happens inside their heads, deciding on many matters to do with the safe and effective use of medicines. In light of this, it is understandable that a study in the Waikato region of New Zealand in 2010, found the public's perception was that pharmacists are 'pill counters' as media stories involving pharmacists usually depict staff counting pills (a task usually done by technicians.)

To get some idea of how your community pharmacist can help you with your health, we will now consider the key roles they play. Obviously, they dispense prescriptions, which involves many more steps than most realise, including legibility, legality, error correction, appropriate dose and quantity, quality and dealing with interactions with medicines, food and supplements.

Prescriptions can involve much time co-ordinating supplies, especially when bureaucratic rules are involved. For instance, a patient discharged from hospital may need a 'Special Authority approval number,' before the government will subsidise certain medicines. Where no application has been submitted, or where it has been rejected, pending more information, pharmacists end up in the invidious position of having to deal with patients who expect supply, yet are not prepared to pay for what is (at the time) an unsubsidised, private prescription.

One key role is to record allergies, even though some patients think this is the sole domain of doctors. I have seen a number of occasions where doctors prescribed medicines to which patients were allergic. In one case, an elderly patient took umbrage when I provided him with an information sheet about an antibiotic prescribed for him. Because his son was a doctor (in another country), somehow, he felt he did not need my help.

Fortunately, he read the information when he got home, and discovered the medicine was one to which he was allergic. He rang and thanked us for our help, whereby we arranged a new prescription from his doctor. Other key roles include:

- Ongoing vigilance for medical problems like someone regularly buying an antacid for an upset stomach, when they should see a doctor to exclude serious problems like stomach cancer, or chronic reflux that could lead to throat cancer.
- Providing comprehensive health and nutrition information to individuals and groups.
- Providing child-safety caps, as necessary.
- Organising destruction of unused medicines.
- Referring patients to support agencies.
- Continually looking for ways to ensure patients adhere to treatment, discussed below.

How well do you take your medicine?

Compliance has been a term used to describe how well a patient complies with a doctor's treatment. As it has overtones of subservience, it has been replaced with the term, adherence. The consequences of not taking medicines as per instructions include illness, hospitalisation, economic costs like medicine wastage, lost work and transmission of infections to others. Poor adherence to treatment is a major problem. A study in the UK found just a third of repeat prescriptions were uncollected.

The World Health Organization (WHO) suggests half of patients on long-term treatment do not take their medicine properly, according to the following categories:

- Patient issues, e.g. arthritis and difficulty opening containers.

- Social issues, e.g. cost and number of doses per day.
- Quality of the relationship between patients and health professionals, e.g. cases where a prescription did not contain a medicine, normally prescribed, and the patient assumed the doctor had ceased it, without any discussion. This can happen when nurses print prescriptions for doctors to sign without patient records, where medicines prescribed at other times, may be over-looked. Clearly, patients need to confirm any prescription alteration is intentional, as do pharmacists dispensing prescriptions.

In my experience, some patients look for reasons to stop taking their medicine, usually because of things they do not know or understand. In some cases, doctors bow to pressure, when others are reluctant, because they fear the real or imagined consequences of their actions.

I recall many a case where patients said something like, "My doctor says my blood pressure is good, so I have stopped taking my pills." Unfortunately, what they failed to understand was that their blood pressure was only controlled when they took their medicine.

When considering whether they should take a medicine, I have seen many patients take more notice of neighbours, family or friends than health professionals. A common example involves the medicine prednisone where lay 'experts' know all the reasons not to take it, but lack any knowledge of benefits, that could even be lifesaving.

To counter the problem, I emphasise that the medicine is like cortisol, a hormone the body makes to control inflammation. Sometimes we need to boost levels, usually for short periods. When patients understand this, they are more likely to take it according to instructions. This is especially important when weaning off it after a long period of treatment, because the body has reduced its production of cortisol and needs time to build up levels again. Stopping suddenly may cause a serious relapse.

When talking to patients, it is important that health professionals appreciate how a patient's worldview can impact how they interpret situations. For example, I once heard a pharmacist express frustration with a patient who had not told her doctor she was not taking her medicine because 'It is not natural.' Clearly, the patient believed she had a good reason for her actions. In another example, I have seen patients on diuretic medicines (to increase urine output) try to counteract the effect and inconvenience, by reducing their fluid intake.

Medicine waste

Taxes in New Zealand subsidise prescription medicines to the tune of $700 million each year. Throughout my working life, I have seen countless examples of money wasted on medicines and seen many ways this can be reduced.

One example was a woman prescribed paracetamol for pain by her doctor. On a home visit, I noticed a stockpile in her cupboard. When asked why she kept getting repeats, she said, "I didn't want anyone to know I was not taking what doctor had ordered, and didn't have the courage to tell him."

Some doctors write prescriptions naively believing patients will follow orders, when they need to spend time building relationships with patients to see their point of view, so they can prescribe accordingly, and reduce waste.

In New Zealand most medicines are subsidised through Pharmac, where the standard cost to the patient is $5, for three months' supply, a fraction of the cost. Some say the fee is not high enough to get people to appreciate the value, when it poses a barrier to others.

Pharmacists can improve adherence to recommended medicine treatment, in many ways, including:

- Counselling patients (ideally in a private area and employing user-friendly language) to ensure they understand key points about their medicine(s). We found it helpful to provide a 'Medication and Supplement Record Card,' including dose, time to take, reason for use etc.

- Tracking repeat collection patterns, where a charge may deter patients collecting repeats they don't want, or need.

- Following up on patients to find out how they're coping with new medicines etc.

- Supplying electronic devices to tell patients what medicine to take, and when.

- Supplying pillboxes, bearing in mind professional issues to consider, including stability of medicines in such containers that are often not airtight, accuracy of loading, labelling and loader accountability. If you take a number of medicines, ask your pharmacist to provide them in professional, hygienic and safe blister packs. You may even qualify to have this service subsidised by the government.

- Reviewing a patient's history on their computer before dispensing, to ensure no duplications, interactions, etc., occur, i.e. not just 'dispensing' medicines according to labels generated from a computer by a technician.

Doctors should ensure the most practical dosage regimen is used. I recall a case where a patient was prescribed a thyroxine tablet three times a day. When dispensing her prescription, I mentioned it was long-acting and usually taken once a day.

Her response was, "Actually I usually forget to take the night time dose." She admitted her doctor did not know this. She was new to me, but records showed her prescriptions lasted longer than they should have, something previous health professionals should have noticed.

Can you see how this sort of situation leads to complications? For example, if this patient went to hospital, staff would give the dose as per the label on the bottle, or the doctor's incorrect record.

Patient safety and choice

A friend asked me why the label on his medicine for leg cramps said 'Do not stop taking.' I explained that many medicines have multiple uses and in his case the instructions were more appropriate for one of its other uses, i.e. depression.

This example highlights the benefits of having a diagnosis, for each medicine on prescriptions. It would enable pharmacists to give patients appropriate advice and alert them to alternatives. (In this case, a magnesium deficiency might be one cause.)

It would also minimise situations where a hospital nurse phoned to chastise me saying, "The label says take two aspirin four times a day, when the patient only takes half a tablet each day for his heart." I explained that the doctor had ordered it that way, probably to save the patient money and time getting repeat prescriptions.

Situations where pharmacists dispense repeat prescriptions from records on a computer, without looking at a prescription, are potentially dangerous. Overseas systems, where patients present a copy of the original prescription, when collecting repeats, are worth consideration.

On the subject of repeats, in some countries, new prescriptions for a medicine automatically cancel previous prescriptions. This avoids potentially dangerous situations where patients 'control' supply of their medicines by telling doctors, nurses or pharmacists 'what they need,' based on outstanding repeats, etc.

Our pharmacy was not busy enough to support two pharmacists, so I had to work through each day, without a break. In the interests of patient safety and sanity, sole pharmacists should be able to take a lunch break, as permitted in the UK. However, the Pharmaceutical Society of New Zealand rejected my request to consider the idea, suggesting I employ a locum pharmacist, which was not economically feasible, or practical.

In June 2011, the Ministry of Health raised concerns about serious adverse reactions and overdoses with paracetamol in children. The liquid form remains one of the most commonly used medicines for minor illnesses in children. Its availability in two strengths increases the risk of confusion and errors, especially when doctors prescribe large bottles for a number of children in a family. A single-strength formula might be safer.

Pharmac has done a good job containing medicine costs since its formation in 1993. However, the job has been relatively easy because it operates with monopolistic control, outside the Commerce Act. A substantial part of their cost containment has been through generic medicines and their 'sole supply' policy, whereby companies compete against each other, with price being a key driver. The result is that medicine costs in New Zealand are generally low, with a plethora of changing brands, creating confusion amongst patients and health providers alike.

My guess is that at least 80% of all prescriptions dispensed in New Zealand are for 'sole supply' medicines fairly often involving bulk containers of loose tablets and capsules, with no patient information leaflets. Some do not even have unique markings, to confirm identity when repacked or mislabelled. Not only does dispensing from these bulk containers take more time, it leads to patients being blasé about little white pills in plastic bottles.

It also causes financial loss to pharmacists when they have not used the balance before the expiry date, which is often short, due to New Zealand being towards the end of the global supply chain. Compensation for such situations seems reasonable.

Ideally, in today's world, all solid dose medicines should be supplied in quality, hygienic 'unit-of-use' blister packs to improve patient adherence to treatment; improve hygiene, safety and reduce the risks of child overdosing. These packs should contain consumer information leaflets and be marked with days of the week, to make it easy for patients to see if they have taken their medicine on the right day etc.

Packs like this also make dispensing safer, as no transfer of medicines from one container to another occurs, and the pharmacist can see the identity, strength and expiry date on the pack, right up to handing it to the patient. Harmonisation of labelling, etc., so we can tap into the Australian market, where these packs are commonly used, would be a great step forward.

Medicines supplied in containers with standard colours and label and packaging style can easily lead to dispensing errors, with serious consequences. To make matters worse, some even have an acronym of their company name as part of their brand names. In the interests of public safety, Pharmac should exclude companies that do this from contracts.

With Pharmac sourcing cheap, overseas medicines and WHO warning of a growing incidence of counterfeit ones, authorities, patients and professionals need to be vigilant.

Over my career, I have seen cases of doctors not complying with prescription laws that may have put patients at risk. Examples include pressuring pharmacists to accept verbal prescriptions from nurses, when this is illegal; false directions on prescriptions so patients get more than the system allows; not providing directions for medicine usage; and using medicines for diseases not approved by authorities.

In the interests of public safety, we need an anonymous reporting system, with power, to ensure results, and protection for whistle-blowers. Doctors violating protocols has prompted moves in the USA for details of prescribing to be monitored.

There was a time when Pharmac replaced a commonly used asthma inhaler with one that easily blocked up and contained alcohol, but reversed the decision following public complaints. Then they replaced an angina spray with one that was bulkier, so less convenient to carry in the pocket, and needed the pump primed for it to work, meaning some patients did not get a correct dose. Fortunately, the original model is available again.

Consumers and prescribers should have a choice, especially as some patients are happy to pay extra for a brand they prefer. Pharmac's sole-supply policy takes that choice away. It may also stop patients claiming on insurance, as some policies only cover prescription medicines on the Pharmac list, which is opposite to what most would expect.

"Just because a medicine is not subsidised does not mean the patient goes without," says Pharmac. "They can have it, if they are prepared to pay on a private prescription." This is true. However, when a medicine is not subsidised, the demand often drops to a point where a company stops importing it.

The business side of pharmacy

This section is here to highlight how business frustrations may detract from professional care pharmacists provide, which could affect your health. For instance, in New Zealand they cannot claim government payment for prescriptions until they are collected. While this seems logical, situations where a patient orders a repeat but does not collect it, or a prescription is faxed to a pharmacy in error, meaning pharmacists are not paid for some work they do, not to mention financial implications when more medicines are ordered, because stock is 'tied up,' waiting for collection that does not eventuate.

In addition, pharmacists are in private business and should be able to charge extra, if the government subsidy is inadequate to cover professional services rendered, just as doctors do.

While people would not expect a supermarket to stock rarely sold products, some patients have trouble understanding why pharmacies do the same. Even if supplied previously, there is no guarantee a medicine will be required again, as the patient may stop taking it, change locations, etc. If you are on a medicine in this category, give your pharmacist appropriate notice, so they can procure more for you.

In a busy pharmacy, prescription errors like a missing signature may be accidentally overlooked, but paid for by the government, in the normal way. However, if an audit detects an error, the pharmacy loses the payment. In one case a pharmacy dispensed a bundle of prescriptions for expensive injections. Three were unsigned, resulting in the pharmacist losing $2,400, even though the doctor later signed the prescriptions, and they were resubmitted. Before electronic-claiming, pharmacists sent prescriptions to a 'pricing office' for payment, where those that were incomplete were returned for completion, and resubmission. The change altered the process, but did not retain 'good faith' principles.

We're all aware of the perils of putting all our eggs in one basket. In my experience, Pharmac's sole-supply policy did this, meaning there was no back-up alternatives so pharmacists ended up juggling stock amongst patients when medicines were out of stock or recalled. Hopefully things have improved.

There have even been times when the situation was so bad Pharmac had to bring back de-listed brands, because the replacement did not work as well as expected, with significant time lags, extra work, frustration and possible patient risk.

Spin-doctors have had a field day espousing Pharmac's virtues. However, a significant amount of the success arises from pharmacies. They have sustained lost income, low morale, amalgamations, closures and a great deal of extra, unpaid work, dealing with ever-changing rules, prices, brands, bulk packs etc., and prescriptions not complying with those rules. On top of this, pharmacy staff spend many hours of unpaid time communicating details of changes to a public that is not always receptive.

Ironically, on 20th May 2005, the Controller and Auditor General released a 45-page report on three-months-at-once-dispensing, which criticised a number of Pharmac's suggestions of savings, but completely ignored the damage done to community pharmacy. A long-overdue study (mid 2013) has commenced to assess the impact of some of Pharmac's policies.

Long term conditions (LTC) pharmacy services

In the past, pharmacy payment has been on a 'fee for service' basis for dispensing prescriptions with the right medicine, in the right dose, at the right time and intervening on innumerable times to improve patient care, correcting doctors' errors, and possibly even saving lives. This simple method of payment has endured for a long time, probably because it was easy for administrators to calculate.

To appreciate some issues surrounding the system, consider the case of a woman who had antibiotic eye drops prescribed for her child. The label on the packet simply said 'Instil three times a day.' Now pharmacists are professionals and, as such, are obliged under the Health and Disability Act in New Zealand, to 'add value' to the dispensing process. This is fine in theory, as long as they are paid adequately, so they don't take shortcuts, which is what happened in this case.

In an ideal world the label should be on the container as many patients tend to discard packets. (In some cases, this is not practical, e.g. some inhaler mouthpieces need washing regularly, to ensure they do not block.) The eye drop label should have specified how many drops (usually a single drop is adequate) and indicated an interval, e.g., every eight hours, to give good coverage. The label should also have given a duration of treatment (typically two days after the eye is clear, i.e. back to normal).

Most pharmacists do much more than basic 'dispensing,' so the $5 they have been getting for a number of years is pitiful. On top of this, District Health Boards let pharmacists renew their dispensing contracts on 1st April 2003, even though CEOs knew of Pharmac's plans to get many medicines dispensed in three-month lots, not monthly. Pharmac calculated a reduction of each pharmacy's annual income of $60,000, with an estimated $24,000 worth of wasted medicines, per pharmacy, per annum.

Ironically, in the past, health administrators had touted the benefits of dispensing medicines monthly so that pharmacists could keep an eye on how well patients took their medicines, etc.

In 2013 the government introduced an experimental system called LTC 'long-term condition, pharmacy service'. It provides a process whereby patients, who need help managing their medicines, get together with their pharmacist to see if they qualify. If they do, the government pays the pharmacist, in a type of 'bulk funding' system.

To give you some idea, consider the case of a patient enrolled in the LTC system. As is required, the pharmacist got the patient to show all her medicines and noticed a stockpile of a medicine to manage cholesterol, to be taken at night, for best effect. The patient took her morning medicines regularly, but tended to forget the night one. Seeing this, the pharmacist arranged for her doctor to change the medicine to one suitable for taking in the morning, along with her other medicines. Now all is well.

Just as some doctors say, their current payment is inadequate to give patients appropriate attention, the LTC system must ensure adequate payment, so pharmacists can do their job in a safe and professional manner, for the benefit of patients.

However, some pharmacists say the LTC formula is so complicated it is virtually impossible to know what payments will be and how long they will take, so business planning is difficult. This is unfortunate, given the savings the government has made, cutting medicine costs over a number of years and the contribution pharmacy has made to this.

If LTC is a success, it will give pharmacists an opportunity to play a greater role in managing peoples' health, as they trained to do, and alleviation of some of the issues raised here. Importantly, the system should address adequate reimbursement for dispensing for patients not classified as LTC.

When all is said and done, pharmacists are highly trained, regularly come near the top of public trust surveys, and are in close contact with the public, so are in an ideal position to be included in public health initiatives, like screening for high blood pressure, as is done in the UK. By now, I trust you appreciate pharmacists do far more than most realise, filling in the gaps after patients leave doctors' surgeries, and you can now see better ways to utilise them and what you can do to help them.

CHAPTER 11

Nutritional Building Blocks

In the *Green Smoothie Revolution*, Victoria Boutenko discusses the emergence of diseases like scurvy, rickets and pellagra a century ago, following industrialisation of food processing, which resulted in the consumption of food, depleted of essential nutrients, with thousands dying, through malnourishment. Because the connection between disease and nutrition was not fully appreciated, the medical profession turned to medicinal drugs for answers.

Some would say not much has changed since then. For instance, Elson M. Haas MD, author of a textbook (USA), *Staying Healthy with Nutrition* (2006) quotes a professor of medicine as saying, "Young doctors are not taught enough nutrition." To add to this, not long ago, there was a story in a local newspaper, reporting a doctor as saying, "I don't generally discuss nutrition with patients, as I hope they already know enough."

Given the magnitude of evidence for the negative impact of poor nutrition, these statements are astounding, especially as my experience is that many people, including some health professionals, don't understand what a healthy lifestyle is.

Now, take a couple of minutes to answer true (T) or false (F) to the following quiz:

1. Hippocrates, the founding father of medicine said, 'Let food be your medicine.'
2. Too many people are eating too many, highly refined carbohydrates, like white flour.
3. Some fats and oils contain bad trans-fatty acids.
4. Soil deficiencies can cause foods to lack nutrients.
5. Good nutrition reduces disease, extends life and repairs damaged cells.

If you answered true to all of them, congratulations you are right!

Whilst not myself a nutritionist, I have, in the course of my research, come across some key points you need to know, to see the big picture. Consult experts for further information and remember food and water are as much elements of care as medicines and operations. With this in mind, let's consider some basics.

Living things are based on molecules containing the chemical carbon, represented by the symbol C. Nutrition involves a multitude of molecules and biochemical processes, derived from a number of nutrients, just as the

26 letters of the alphabet open the door to tens of thousands of words. Our body lets nutrients in and toxins out, in a process involving about 25 million cells per day.

Below is a brief description of the main nutrients. The calculations are for a 2000-calorie (8,370kJ) intake, typical for an average adult female. [65]

Minerals

Nearly everyone has heard about the macro-minerals such as calcium, magnesium, phosphorus, potassium and sodium that occur in relatively large amounts in our bodies. What is less well known is the important role of trace minerals, also known as trace elements or micro-minerals, present in small amounts. Think of them as spark plugs to kick-start biochemical functions.

Some are essential for a healthy life, meaning we need to get them from the environment, i.e. boron, copper, cobalt, chromium, iodine, iron, manganese, molybdenum, selenium, silicon and zinc. Some are 'probably essential' including lithium, nickel, strontium, tin and vanadium, which highlights that we still have some way to go to fully understand the inter-relationships between biochemistry, health and nutrition.

Vitamins

These are nutrients required only in small amounts to sustain life. Think of them also as spark plugs that get things happening. We discuss the important role of vitamins, in more detail, later.

Bioflavonoids, polyphenols, carotenoids, fats, oils, fibre and water are all discussed in specific sections to come.

Carbohydrates

Also known as 'carbs,' they are organic compounds of carbon, hydrogen and oxygen from plants, produced by a process called photosynthesis. They are a source of energy and include common sugar. Complex, long chain carbohydrates, known as polysaccharides contain up to 10,000 molecules of simple sugars.

Foods contain different kinds of carbohydrates, e.g. starchy carbs, that tend to break down easily into sugar and are found in foods such as carrots, potatoes, squash, bananas and grains; and non-starchy carbs, found in green leafy vegetables.

Whilst some suggest the WHO recommendation of 2014 are too high, at least restrict simple sugars to less than 5% (typically, half a can of soft drink) of your energy needs and total carb intake to 60% e.g. 300g being 60% of

2000 calories divided by 4 as there are 4 calories (17kJ) per g (gram). [www.cph.co.nz]

Protein

The sources of protein include animals, grains, nuts, seeds, legumes and some green leafy vegetables, broken down in the body into amino acids, that provide 17kJ (4cal)/g of energy and muscle. Aim for about 0.8g/kg per day. The amount of protein in foods varies, e.g. 1/3 cup of nuts equals 10g; 100g of red or white meat equals 25g, and 100g of fish equals 16g. Too much protein can lead to kidney damage (especially with low water intake), heart disease and accelerated ageing.

Air

We need air for oxygen and should deep breathe on a regular basis for good health.

Sunlight

This not only helps to relax the body, it is also a prime source of Vitamin D, discussed later.

Enzymes and digestion

We have no teeth in our stomachs, a fact to remind us to chew food thoroughly, down to about the size of half a grain of rice. The body's enzymes can then easily break it down for use.

Proteases break proteins down to amino acids; lipases break fats down to glycerol, and fatty acids, and amylases break carbohydrates (starches) down to simple sugars, i.e. sugar (sucrose or cane sugar) is broken down to glucose and fructose.

Specific enzymes, like lactase, break down milk sugar (lactose) into glucose and galactose. Lacking this enzyme will make you intolerant to dairy products. Ptyalin in the mouth helps to break down carbohydrates, especially with thorough chewing, or swilling, before swallowing. Some fruits like Kiwifruit tenderise meat through enzyme action. Some suggest drinking water during a meal dilutes enzymes and reduces their efficacy.

Our stomach acid has a number of important functions including: aiding digestion; absorption of most minerals, protein and vitamin B12; and protecting us from gut infections.

Typically, orthodox practitioners treat stomach conditions like indigestion with medicines to reduce stomach acid levels, which can increase the risk of hospital-acquired pneumonia (HAP). Some may also reduce mineral absorption, i.e. there might be an association with low calcium and osteoporosis and deficiencies of important minerals like selenium.

I discussed this with a medical research doctor and he laughed, saying 'it wasn't proven.' I then suggested this would be a good research project for him, but he showed no interest. Following the discussion, I spoke with a local laboratory technologist and discovered requests to test mineral levels were low. I also discovered that in 2011 the FDA recognized that low magnesium levels could be caused by these medicines.

Stomach acid levels also tend to drop with age, generally halving from age 30 to age 60. Other causes include excess food, zinc deficiency, chemical toxicity, stress and diseases including candidiasis (thrush), parasites, multiple sclerosis, arthritis, autoimmune disorders, stomach cancer and coeliac disease.

Fats and oils

Often maligned, fats and oils, also known as lipids, are an important part of our cells, hormones and nerves. In general, fats are solid, and oils are liquid, at room temperature, insoluble in water and act as an 'energy storage' system. They contain twice the energy of the same weight of carbohydrate, provide insulation in the skin and around some vital organs and add flavour to food. They can suppress the appetite by slowing down the passage of food through the digestive tract and increase the absorption of some nutrients i.e. lycopene from tomatoes.[66] [67] We classify fats and oils (chains of fatty acids) as follows:

Saturated fats

Chemically, saturated fats have an acid group at one end, attached to a chain of carbon atoms, saturated with hydrogen atoms. They are a component of cell membranes in our body. Meat, dairy, coconut and palm oil are key sources.

Mono-unsaturated fatty acids (MUFA)

These have one (mono) double bond. They lower total and LDL (lousy) cholesterol, with little effect on the HDL (healthy) cholesterol. Avocado, macadamia nut and olive oil are some sources.

Poly-unsaturated fatty acids (PUFA)

These consist of chains with more than one double bond and are more susceptible to oxidation than mono-unsaturated oils.

Omega-6 fatty acids (O6)

A group of unsaturated fatty acids that contain more than one double bond, no closer than six carbons from the methyl end of the molecule, prevalent in the oils of seeds and grains, like sunflower and corn oil. They are essential for health, with some being found to lower total and LDL cholesterol. However, too high an intake could lower healthy HDL cholesterol and cause inflammation.

Other sources include meat, nuts, safflower, soya bean, grape seed oil and canola oil, and some natural and some genetically modified rapeseed. To date, a number of small-scale studies suggest canola oil has a beneficial effect on LDL cholesterol and heart health.

A UK review found it is high in mono-unsaturated fatty acids (MUFA). Recent advances, using conventional plant breeding, have led to the development of high-oleic canola, which has an increased level of MUFA and greater oxidative stability, making it suitable for a wide range of culinary purposes, including frying.[68]

Super-unsaturated fatty acids

Often referred to as poly-unsaturated fatty acids, omega-3 fatty acids (O3) contain more than one double bond, no closer than three carbon atoms (hence the name) from the methyl end of the molecule. They are not suitable for cooking, as high temperature destroys them.

Healthy individuals should consume 500mg daily of O3 containing EPA (eicosa-pentaenoic acid) and DHA (docosa-hexaenoic acid), but new research is suggesting two to three times this amount, especially for those with heart disease.[69] Some believe adequate intake is important to reduce behavioural and learning problems in children. Its anti-inflammatory effect may be helpful in inflammatory autoimmune diseases like rheumatoid arthritis.

Sources include grass-fed sheep and beef, fish (especially wild and oily, like salmon and sardines), walnuts, cauliflower and eggs. Fish oil supplements are available, when dietary intake is inadequate, but be on the lookout for environmental contaminants like mercury. Recently there has been a move to krill oil. This is a more concentrated source and, because krill are short-lived and are at the bottom of the food chain, are less likely to accumulate toxins, than fish at the top.

Although flaxseed oil contains high amounts of the omega-3 fatty acid, alpha-linolenic acid (ALA, LNA), a poor diet may mean poor conversion to the beneficial DHA and EPA fatty acids.

Ratio of Omega-6 to Omega-3 fatty acids

Before we came to eat processed foods, humans consumed omega-6 and omega-3 fatty acids in roughly equal amounts. Today the ratio is around 20 to 1, which is significant because omega-6 fatty acids tend to be inflammatory, whereas omega-3 fatty acids tend to be anti-inflammatory.

"This issue is more important than the LDL form of cholesterol," says Dr P M Ridker, a US cardiologist.[70] Having said that, a report in 2011 from the American Heart Association says omega-6 may not be as inflammatory as we think and can help reduce heart disease, control blood pressure and decrease insulin resistance.

Trans-fatty acids (TFA)

Most molecules in our bodies occur in the 'cis' format, where chemical branches are on the same side of the carbon chain; whereas in some, such as trans-fatty acids, chemical branches are on opposite 'trans' sides. Trans-fatty acids usually result from manufacturing processes above 160 degrees C. and are bad for health.

They upset the balance between good and bad forms of cholesterol and may be more 'artery-clogging' than saturated fats. Some researchers suggest that some negative ideas about the consumption of saturated fats may have arisen because, from ignorance, older health statistics did not account for TFA.

The countries reported as banning TFAs set upper limits of consumption, e.g. in 2003 the Danish Nutrition Council recommended phasing out of manufactured TFAs in foods. However, if the TFA content in finished food is less than 1g per 100g, the Danes consider the food free of it. USA regulators allow products with less than half a gram per serve be labelled as containing 'no trans fats,' meaning, someone consuming a number of these products in one day may be blissfully ignorant of the danger.

In 2007, the New York City Council was so concerned about TFAs that it banned them in restaurant food and now the FDA plans to ban them outright. TFA content in foods in New Zealand is only required if the supplier makes nutritional content claims in their marketing. WHO recommends no more than 1% daily intake from TFAs, i.e. for a 2,000cal (8,368kJ) intake this equals 20cal (83.7kJ) or 2.2g. Fats and oils provide 38 kJ (9cal)/g.)

Food Standards Australia and New Zealand (FSANZ) say the average for New Zealanders is well below this, but we are still getting around 14-16% of our daily kilojoules from TFAs and saturated fats combined, well above the recommendations of no more than 10%.

Partial hydrogenation occurs in the production of a wide range of processed foods, especially those that are baked and fried, so may contain TFAs and altered fat substances. These include pies, biscuits (cookies), breakfast cereals, cakes, fried chicken (especially with the skin on), margarines, commercial oils, mayonnaises, corn chips, potato chips, dips and toppings, doughnuts and salad dressings. Be on the lookout for other terms used to disguise them.

General fat/oil issues

Aim for a fat intake of 30% of energy in the following ratios (numbers in brackets are the weight recommended for a 2000-calorie intake): about 5% (11g) poly-unsaturated, 15% (33g) mono-unsaturated, 10% (22g) saturated fat and minimal, or zero, trans-fatty acids. Oils need less than 20% saturated fat to get a New Zealand Heart Foundation tick.

The jury is still out on saturated fats. For more information, see www.eatforkeeps.com. Also, whilst researchers say more data is needed to assess the effects of fats replacing the saturated ones, a meta-analysis in 2010 reported in the March issue of the *American Journal of Clinical Nutrition*, found no difference in the incidence of heart disease and strokes in people on high and low intakes of saturated fat, from natural sources.

Consider lemon juice, balsamic vinegar and extra-virgin olive oil, as alternatives to manufactured salad dressings that may contain lots of sugar. Avocado and hummus can be natural alternatives to butter etc. When buying oil - consider the taste, what you will use it for and how healthy it is. No single oil meets all needs.

Do not fry your food regularly, as this causes potentially dangerous oxidative stress. Use moderate heat (less than 160 deg. C) when cooking with fats and oils. High smoke point oils, often referred to as refined, bleached and deodorised (RBD) oils are for 'occasional' high-heat cooking. They include peanut, soybean, canola and rice bran. Some have high concentrations of omega-6 fatty acids that may contribute to inflammation.

Butter goes bright yellow when oxidised, so be careful about the setting of the conditioner in your refrigerator to reduce this. Alternatively, blend with oil and freeze for easier spreading once thawed.

Use vegetable oils that are fresh and stored in a cool, dark place, to reduce oxidation and rancidity, which brings on an unpleasant fishy (turpentine) taste or smell. Ideally use within a month or two of opening.

The TV show Fair Go in May 2012 showed a significant number of brands of olive oil on New Zealand supermarket shelves failed a sensory test and some failed a chemical test. Most were from overseas, highlighting the need to be vigilant, especially as it's not always possible to recognise rancid oil. Suppliers have challenged the results and the quality of the testing, so the story is ongoing.

Fibre

Fibre, consisting mostly of long chain polysaccharides is a generic term for the components of plant cell walls, sometimes called roughage, or cellulose. Fruit, vegetables, legumes, oat-bran, greens, peels, nuts, seeds, and whole grains are some good sources. The outside parts generally contain more fibre than the inside, therefore, milling of grains and unnecessary peeling of fruits and vegetables removes a significant percentage.

Experts suggest we need about 25g of fibre per day, yet most get much less than this. You can check if you are getting enough by noting the length of your bowel motion. Ideally, it should be about 300mm long.[71] Countries like the USA and Germany have toilet bowl shapes that make it easy to do this.

Fibre is nature's way of sweeping clean your stomach, small intestine and bowel. It removes toxins, allows nutrients to be absorbed, and slows the rate sugars are absorbed, by slowing the movement of food through the system. It also lowers LDL cholesterol and helps reduce bowel cancer rates.

The ideal transit time from stomach to bowel movement is 12 to 24 hours. One way to check is to drink a quarter of a cup of beetroot juice, and note the time it takes to colour your faeces. However, if you're dehydrated, or have low amounts of fibre in your food, transit times tend to be longer.

Regarding constipation, you should always consult a health professional before resorting to chronic (long-term) stimulant laxative use, as this can lead to situations where the bowel muscles will not work without them. Laxatives with different modes of action are preferable. Extra fibre may help, but beware of blockages especially if you are dehydrated.

CHAPTER 12

Food is Your Foundation

Food supplies our bodies with the nutritional building blocks needed to be healthy. Before refrigeration and speedy transport, most of what was available depended on the seasons, what grew locally and what was available from trading and hunting.

Unlike carnivore cats that would starve amongst fruit and vegetables, most humans are omnivores, eating meat and plants.

In different parts of the world people are genetically different and eat different foods. Some eat often and heartily and do not gain weight, while others seem to pack on extra kilos walking through the kitchen. Differences can even be observed within the same family, where one sibling is overweight, hungry all the time and lethargic, and the other is skinny and hyperactive. Clearly, nature and nurture play their roles, right down to foods switching genes on or off.

Anthropologists and other scientists use the term 'diet' to describe the different foods people eat, whereas typically it describes weight loss programs. Regardless of the terms used, the key factor is to understand diet and healthy eating as meaning the same thing, i.e. something to do all the time.

Traditional eating habits

It is valuable to look at the traditional eating habits of healthy races around the world, to see what we can learn and apply to our own nutrition. One person to do this in the 1930s was Dr Weston A. Price, who published his results in *Nutrition and Physical Degeneration.*

At one end of the scale, he found healthy Inuits on a traditional diet of seal meat (80% protein and fat) and fish, and with low levels of heart disease and cancer. At the other extreme, he found incredibly healthy tribes in Africa, predominately eating grains.[72]

Other traditional diets include the Mediterranean diet, associated with good health, with a focus on fruit, vegetables, legumes (peas, beans), nuts, unprocessed cereals, garlic, extra virgin olive oil, white meat including fish, moderate dairy, red wine with red meat eaten sparingly.

In some traditional diets considered healthy, all the edible parts of some animals are eaten, including the liver and heart.

Close inspection of the traditional French diet reveals some key health factors, e.g. smaller portions, no seconds, no snacks between meals and long and leisurely eating sessions with a focus on social interaction and enjoyment.

If we look at the ancient Indian practice of Ayurvedic medicine, we find its followers mostly ate fruit and vegetables, high quality carbohydrates (wholegrain bread and wholegrain pasta) and legumes, with a focus on fats from fish, olive oil, avocados and nuts.

Most traditional Asian diets are associated with health and longevity, e.g. in the Okinawa region in Japan we find low death rates from heart disease, with a lifestyle that focuses on serenity, daily exercise, low saturated fats, generous amounts of fruit and vegetables, soy protein and fish.

Metabolic typing diet

Following on from the work of Dr Price, W. Wolcott and T. Fahey describe in *The Metabolic Typing Diet,* a system to determine what eating plan (diet) is ideal for you.[73] Basically you answer 65 questions, including: personality, how temperature affects you, health issues like signs of cracking skin, and foods you prefer, e.g. how do you feel if you eat meat for breakfast, what is your reaction to sour foods like pickles, and what kinds of food bring your energy levels down. Your answers, analysed, put you in one of three groups, as follows (percentages are just a guide):

The **protein type diet** consists of 70% protein and fats, and 30% carbohydrates. Avoid alcohol, allergenic foods, caffeine, fruit juices, citrus fruits, sugar, high GI/GL foods and foods high in phalates and oxalic acid (discussed below) and gluten.

The **carbohydrate type diet** consists of 60% carbohydrates and 40% protein and fats. Avoid alcohol, caffeine, sugar, high-fat foods, foods high in purines (organ meats, pate, beef and chicken liver) and thyroid-suppressing, cruciferous vegetables, like cabbage, cauliflower, broccoli, etc.

The **mixed type diet** consists of half carbohydrates and half protein and fats. Avoid alcohol, caffeine, sugar, fruit juices and foods high in oxalic acid.

It is important to involve the appropriate health professionals to guide and monitor you. Trial and error are encouraged to fine-tune eating plans.

Phytates

Phytates (salts of phytic acid) are chemicals in the bran portion of grains and the skins of legumes. Wheat, oats and soy contain the highest levels. They bind with minerals like calcium, iron, magnesium, zinc and phosphorus in the intestine and when consumed to excess can cause intestinal upset, mineral deficiency and bone loss. Soaking, heating, sprouting and fermenting lowers phytate levels in food. Sourdough bread, with a long fermentation process, is almost entirely phytate-free.

Oxalates

Oxalates (salts of oxalic acid) interfere with the absorption of minerals like calcium, iron, magnesium and zinc and can cause kidney stones. They occur in a variety of foods including, black tea, blackberry, beets, chocolate, cocoa, cranberries, red currants, endive, gooseberries, grapes, green peppers, plums, raspberries, rhubarb, strawberries and tomatoes. The body manufactures oxalic acid and cooking destroys it, so dietary intake is not usually an issue, unless consuming massive quantities.[74]

Wholefoods

Most experts focus on eating fresh, unprocessed (unchanged) food. Whilst most people understand the wholefood concept regarding fruits and vegetables, some struggle with issues around grains, which are small, hard cereal seeds that include buckwheat, barley, maize, millet, oats, rice, rye, spelt, triticale, wheat and quinoa.

Components are the central core, called the endosperm, which makes up 80% of the seed, composed primarily of starch and proteins. The germ portion (3% - 5%) comprises the future sprouting potential and most concentrated part, and the bran (15%), is the outer covering, composed primarily of indigestible cellulose, or fibre.

Focus on eating wholegrains that confer health benefits in many conditions including plaque build-up in arteries, congestive heart failure, high blood pressure, Type 2 diabetes, insulin resistance, obesity and weight gain, rather than the refined grains, where processing usually involves removal of the germ and bran components.[75] Opt for wholegrain varieties of breads, breakfast cereals and pastas and sprouted or fermented grain products like sourdough bread.

Methods that retain the endosperm, bran, germ and vitamins in their natural, original proportions with minimal heating in the processing are ideal, e.g. stone grinding.

Consider sprouting your own seeds to bring out the vitamins and minerals, e.g. mung beans, using a jar with a stainless steel mesh lid for drainage.

Organic food

Organic farming combines scientific knowledge and technology with ecology. Essentially it involves natural biological processes to achieve sustainability and harmony between the soil, microbes, earthworms, insects, plants and animals.

Key factors include soil testing, manures, composting, biological pest control and mechanical cultivation. A typical example would be legumes to fix nitrogen into the soil, cows grazing a section of land, followed by free-range hens, and goats to control gorse. Natural insect predators are encouraged with crop rotation to confuse pests and renew the soil. Whilst conventional agriculture uses synthetic pesticides and fertilisers, organic farmers use natural varieties.

Some farmers who have changed from conventional (chemical) farming to organic farming recognised the benefits, but also felt ostracised (isolated) from the local community 'because they were different.' Fonterra, New Zealand's dairy co-operative, responsible for approximately 30% of the world's dairy exports, say they are working towards being more organic, with demand outstripping production.

With the emergence of grand scale, industrialised agriculture servicing large concentrations of populations around the world, organic food may be produced at very long distances from the markets they supply, which could affect the quality. In some countries, production companies are so big they will not deal with local producers who, even though they may produce great product, cannot meet the volumes demanded.

In light of this, it is great to see the growing support for local farmers' markets and high profile celebrities like Michelle Obama emphasising the benefits of growing your own produce at home or in community gardens, with a biological focus including composting and worm farms.

On one side of the fence, we have the protagonists of organic food, claiming a more natural, less toxic, tastier and healthier product, and on the other side the antagonists challenging the claims and even suggesting 'organic' is too general a term and needs to be clearly defined in law. Some consumers claim organic foods are expensive, yet chef, Jamie Oliver argues that conventional economy ranges are cut-price, lower quality and bad value. He says, "If we witnessed how most meat is produced, many of us would become vegetarian."[76]

Resolving the issues is difficult, due to gaps in our knowledge about health and nutrition, costs, validity of tests etc.[77]

Cooked or raw?

Cooking includes baking, barbecuing, boiling, steaming, frying, grilling (broiling), slow cooking and microwaving. It can destroy toxins and harmful microbes, so long as the temperature and duration are adequate, as discussed in the hygiene section.

Unfortunately, heat may also destroy vitamins and good bacteria such as lactobacillus acidophilus; enzymes important for digestion, and carotenoids - a family of over 700 naturally occurring colourful pigments found in fruit and vegetables (associated with a lower risk of diseases like cancer), leading to what some describe as 'dead' food.

Knowing some researchers say raw broccoli has more anti-cancer properties than cooked broccoli, I encourage the grandchildren to pick it from our garden and enjoy eating 'little green trees.' Interestingly, the *Preventative Medicine Journal* reports child intake of vegetables doubled when carrots were rebranded as 'X-ray vision carrots; beans as 'Silly Dilly green beans' and broccoli as 'tiny tasty tree tops.'

However, heat may modify cell membranes to enhance the digestibility, bioavailability (absorption) and nutrition of some foods, e.g. carrots, legumes and tomatoes. Research at the Chicago Institute of Food Science in 2009 showed no nutritional loss in cooking beetroot, garlic and artichoke. Increased antioxidant levels occurred when celery, carrots, tomatoes and green beans were cooked by all methods.[78] The research also found the highest antioxidant loss in boiled or microwaved cauliflower, boiled peas and boiled or fried zucchini.

Too much heat during cooking can convert fatty acids into altered toxic forms including trans-fatty acids and highly toxic heterocyclic aromatic amines (HAA), strongly linked to some cancers. Researchers have noted a substance called acryl amide is formed when carbohydrate-rich foods are heated, causing plaque build-up, hardening of the arteries and an increased incidence of some cancers.

It seems prudent to minimise high-temperatures, especially when barbecuing, frying, grilling (broiling) and microwaving. Cooking methods that produce smoke and flare-ups may expose us to highly toxic polynuclear aromatic hydrocarbons (PAH), strongly linked to many forms of cancer. [79]

The key here is to think about what food you mostly eat and research the best methods of preparation. Generally, light steaming of vegetables is ideal, so as not to overcook them and affect quality, taste and enjoyment.

Cookware

Concerns circulate about the safety of non-stick cookware. If you use them, take special care not to damage the surface by overheating or scratching. Discard if damaged and clean with a soft cloth, not a brush. A number of brands use Teflon, so check with suppliers for safety information and if you have any concerns, consider alternatives such as ceramic, cast iron, or stainless steel.[80] Leaching of heavy metals from cookware made from aluminium and copper may pose health hazards.

Microwave ovens

The jury is still out on the overall safety of microwaving, with *The Healthy Food Guide* (2011) suggesting there is 'no evidence one way or another.' Russian and German research, reported by US researcher William Kopp provides some key points, as follows.

While the evidence is not entirely clear, microwaves may damage food enzymes, fats, oils and vitamins, and form free radicals. Err on the safe side and think whether you really have to use this method. If so, use as low a power as practical, up to a maximum of 500 watts, about half (50%) the power of most machines.

Some research suggests there is less nutrient loss in microwaved food, compared to conventional cooking, most likely due to shorter heating times.[81] However, there are fears about the microbiological safety of microwaved food, because of the uneven heating. Microwaving seems to retain the nutrients when heating breast milk and infant formula, so long as the temperature is kept below 60 degrees Celsius.

Microwave cooking in plastic containers may be hazardous to your health as the intense heat generated can leach chemicals into the food. If you really have to use plastic, wrap or cover food using a microwave safe product; keep power and exposure time to a minimum. Use glass containers wherever possible.

Real 'living' food

In *Green for Life*, V. Boutenko tells of the lengthy time she spent studying and comparing what chimpanzees and humans eat.[82] She notes we tend to crave sugar, salt and fat, whereas they crave greens and fruit. They have powerful jaws with which to chew their food and rupture it, releasing nutrients.

Changing eating habits has meant humans have lost this ability, so making raw smoothies of different fruits and vegetables is the answer. She says if you try this for a couple of weeks, you will notice how much better you will feel and how much vitality you have.

She also discusses a range of medical benefits: a lessening of wrinkles, a fresher look and improved vision, a wonderful taste in the mouth, better sleep, improved bowel motions, more energy and a loss of cravings for sweet, fatty and salty foods, drugs, caffeine and tobacco.

She also includes a number of recipes. Adapt them to suit yourself, sip slowly, and separate them from other foods by at least 40 minutes. Refrigerate and use within three days and include a variety of greens. A typical recipe is two cups water, two cups green leafy (non-starchy) vegetables, one or two pieces of fruit, some herbs and celery to make about a litre, which is consumed each day, ideally using organic produce.

Slow juicers that do not heat-damage the enzymes in the food are preferable. To emphasise varying nutritional content of vegetables, Ms. Boutenko suggests we group them as follows:

1. Flowers and roots such as carrots, broccoli and potato (but beware of extra carbs in root vegetables.)
2. Non-sweet items such as cucumber and tomato.
3. Green leafy vegetables such as kale, cabbage and lettuce are an excellent source of nutrients, including proteins.

The *Raw for 30 Days* video clip on www.youtube.com demonstrates the medical benefits of raw fruit and vegetables on a group of diabetics, and the award-winning documentary 'Supercharge Me!' features a certified 'live food chef,' highlighting the value of eating some raw foods.[83]

Food quality

Many factors affect produce production including climate, growing conditions, type of fertiliser, whether nutrients are absorbed from the soil or not, right down to the side of a tree on which a crop grows.

Once produced, there are many steps in the movement of food into and out of our lives including harvesting, transportation, storage, preparation and processing, packaging, presentation, purchasing, chewing, digestion, absorption, utilisation in the body and elimination. In this chain of events there are many 'opportunities' for food to be affected, due to the effects of light, heat, moisture, oxygen, microbes and chemical and physical contamination. Quality is dependent on ensuring control of all these factors, a challenging task.

On top of this, we see producers putting profit before the well-being of the consumers, compromising the quality of their food as in the case of melamine in a Chinese dairy factory that made nearly 300,000 babies sick and killed six. Then we had pupils in Auckland discovering that a fruit juice contained no vitamin C, contrary to the label.

Also, more and more sugar is being added to a greater range of processed foods, often without us realizing it. This is happening because it is a cheap source of energy, so the food industry uses it in lieu of more expensive ingredients. The more this happens, the more people buy, according to Professor R. Listig, Paediatric Endocrinologist of the University of California, who says sugar is toxic, damages livers, increases cell-ageing and interferes with the brain's ability to know how much to eat.

Some growers' markets have emerged out of frustrations with supermarkets paying low prices for produce, which may have contributed to poorer quality produce, as suppliers cut corners.

Aflatoxin, is a naturally occurring toxin produced by a mould that grows on corn, rice, wheat, peanuts, almonds, walnuts, sunflower seeds and spices, such as black pepper and coriander.[84] It is considered to be a powerful carcinogen (cancer-causing agent) and linked particularly to liver cancer.[85] Hopefully authorities are keeping a good lookout for it in products like peanut butter.

Produce can appear 'fresh' for a relatively long time, even though it has suffered rapid and significant nutrient loss. Broccoli heads may lose 50-80% of their vital nutrient content between harvest and point of sale.[86] Researchers from Finland say blanching vegetables results in 30% loss of antioxidant content.[87]

A wide range of foods around the world are being produced through genetic modification (GM) including meat, chocolate, milk, corn, fruit, soy, canola oil, corn oil, cottonseed oil and sugar beet. The unknown factor has the public concerned about effects like endocrine disruption, organ damage, decreased fertility, allergies and pesticide resistance.

Processing can provide ways to reduce waste and extend the life of foods, e.g. frozen peas may be just as nutritious as fresh ones, especially if harvested at the peak of condition, snap frozen soon after and temperature-controlled, to point of use. Cans, excluding light and air, are another example.

Freeze-dried strawberries may have more antioxidant activity than fresh fruit. Some say fermentation improves cabbage to produce sauerkraut, with cancer-fighting properties and long storage capabilities.

Sometimes processing involves changes to make food more appealing, e.g., margarine is actually grey, but is coloured yellow, and poultry fed beta-carotene to give the yolks more colour. At other times foods may not be as healthy as we think, e.g. farmed salmon, fed corn, may have less omega-3 fatty acids than grass-fed cows.

Processing may alter the nutritional value of foods, so that foods we perceive as healthy may not be, e.g. most instant noodles are cooked, then deep-fried to remove the water, leaving (possibly bad) fat behind.

Whilst most of us consider yoghurt to be extra healthy, a television show found one brand had the same nutrition as milk. As well as this, the fruit in it was for flavour; there was little fibre, and much of the nutrients were lost in the production process, including the good acidophilus bacteria, especially if more than two weeks old. [88]

Bleached flours may have lowered nutritional value. Functional foods, fortified with nutrients, not from natural sources, may not be ideal.[89] Food production may involve irradiation, especially when imported. Sometimes subtle issues affect quality, e.g. nutritionist Dr N. Barnard, says crushing or dicing onions and garlic ten minutes before cooking activates their nutrients.

Most foods need to be refrigerated, frozen or stored in a cool, dry larder to slow deterioration. If freezing or refrigeration is required, ensure appliances achieve the right temperatures, as discussed under food hygiene. Check with suppliers regarding how best to store their product e.g. some suggest we store eggs in the refrigerator, in their packaging.

Ethylene is an odourless ripening gas produced by fruit and vegetables. Products are now available to place in the refrigerator, to absorb it and extend storage time (shelf life).

Nuts tend to have a short life, hence some experts suggest we keep them in their shell and refrigerate or freeze them, to maintain freshness and nutritional value.

It is encouraging to observe the work the New Zealand government is doing to monitor key areas of our food, including:

- Analysis of sales data.
- Comprehensively monitoring the nutrient content of manufactured foods.
- Monitoring food-marketing practices.
- Investigating the value of additional data collections, such as the diabetes 'Get Checked Aotearoa' collected by doctor groups.
- Analysis of data on nutrition and health status, including socio-demographic and regional inequalities in nutrition, i.e. the New Zealand Total Diet Survey happens every five years.[90]
- Ongoing surveys including the measurement of height and weight in adults and children and their nutrition.
- Improving the co-ordination and dissemination of food and nutrition monitoring data. www.foodsmart.govt.nz

Glycemic Index and Glycemic Load

The Glycemic (Glycaemic) Index (GI) is a means of comparing how quickly foods containing carbohydrates raise blood sugar (glucose) levels. Foods that cause a rapid rise, and an excessive release of insulin are known as 'high glycaemic foods' and those that cause a slower, sustained increase, as shown in the graph below, as 'low-glycaemic foods.' GI calculations, are based on 50g of food. Glucose has a value of 100.

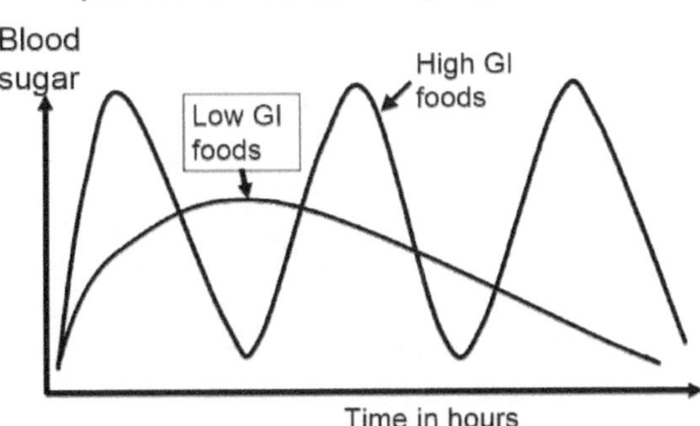

GI is not always reliable, e.g. watermelon has a high GI value, yet is mostly water, containing few calories, so the concept of GL (Glycemic Load) has been developed. This is calculated by multiplying the amount of carbohydrate (g) in a serving by that food's Glycemic Index and dividing that number by 100, i.e. it is based on a portion of food normally eaten at one sitting, rather than 50g used to calculate GI. For an individual food portion, GL 0-10 is low, 11-19 is moderate and over 20 is high.

Healthy eating, focused on lower GI/GL foods, results in less fluctuation in blood sugar levels, less insulin resistance and associated disease including diabetes, obesity and dementia.

Focus on wholegrain products, lentils, non-tropical fruits, nuts and green leafy vegetables and less on sugar, cakes, white bread etc. Tropical fruits generally have higher GI/GL than non-tropical fruits and riper fruit tends to have higher values. Some brown bread is simply coloured white bread. Other key points include:

- Potatoes are a good source of nutrients including vitamin C and potassium. However, GI/GL values vary significantly.

- Different forms of foods may have different values, e.g. one-minute oats have higher values than raw oats. Soaking raw oats overnight reduces cooking time and phytate levels. Consuming a slow digesting, low GI/GL meal such as rolled oats means you're not chasing a snack within a couple of hours, as often happens with many breakfast cereals.

- Some foods lower the GI/GL of other foods, e.g. protein lowers the GI/GL of potatoes if eaten at the same time, and dietary fats suppress the appetite and fluctuations in blood sugars by slowing down the passage of food through the digestive tract.[91]

- Beware: details on some websites may not be specific enough, e.g. is the pasta wholemeal or refined? Also, 'al dente' (lightly cooked) pasta has a lower GI/GL than well-cooked pasta and finely ground grains can have higher values.

- Different data sources may show different values due to different testing methods or simply reflect different batches.

- Brown rice retains the outer bran and germ with a GI value of around 50 in most varieties, whereas some white rice, with the bran and germ removed can have a GI from 50 to 80.

In the final analysis, there is no substitute for checking with manufacturers or websites such as www.glycemicindex.com or www.health.harvard.edu or www.nutritionfoundation.org.nz.

Insulin resistance

Type 2 Diabetes is a form of insulin resistance where the body increases insulin levels in an attempt to overcome the problem.

The Ministry of Health website says, "Eat plenty of breads and cereals, preferably wholegrain and focus on low fat foods," reflecting an idea that emerged years ago that we would curb the rise in obesity if people reduced their fat intake and ate 'plenty of carbohydrates.'

Following this advice, many people have substituted fat with highly processed, high GI/GL carbohydrates leading to insulin resistance, obesity and diabetes where excess carbohydrates convert to fat, because the insulin is not working as well as it should and high insulin levels switch on fat storage mechanisms.

Ignorance about insulin resistance was apparent when the Kentucky Fried Chicken company released a 'Double Down burger,' containing chicken and bacon, but no bun. Suddenly 'experts' were up in arms about the product, claiming it to be unhealthy. In fact, it was lower in kilojoules and fat, had more protein, and was less likely to cause insulin resistance, compared to some burgers on the market.

Welfare and sustainability

We value food for the nutrition it provides, offset by the personal, social, economic and environmental costs of getting it. Most people are fussy about the cars they drive and the clothes they wear, yet do not apply the same standards to their food. Before we delve further into this subject, let's look at some issues surrounding the sources of food.

In *The Omnivore's Dilemma*, Michael Pollan (USA), describes a confined animal feeding operation (CAFO) where farm animals are indoors for their lifetime, and an accelerated growth of livestock reaching the same live weight in three years that took six years in 1950.

Pollan talks about the consequences of this on the welfare of the environment and the quality of food produced, e.g. meat with less omega-3 and more saturated fat than grass-fed animals; and the irony of cows needing antibiotics when the cause may be the environment and feeding them corn, not grass.

To complicate things further there are a host of other issues, including subsidised crops using synthetic fertilisers (produced from oil that has other uses), erosion and soil compaction. Sometimes welfare issues are a secondary consideration, e.g. using palm kernels as a stock feed and justifying this as a 'waste product' from palm oil production. Unfortunately, it's associated with the massive destruction of rainforests, affecting animals such as orang-utans, not to mention the additional pollution and increased transportation costs.

Bio-fuel crops are taking up valuable growing space, when experts say the world is not producing enough food. Recently the price of almonds has climbed, due to a lack of bees in the main growing areas of California.

As a city dweller, I often wonder about stock being kept in paddocks, with little shelter. Interestingly, a New Zealand study found providing shade, to reduce heat stress, led to better grazing, happier cattle, and possibly even better meat.

A TVNZ *Rural Delivery* television series in 2012, suggests cows do not like to be milked early in the morning, as is mostly the case. Because of this, and the fact that it may have a detrimental effect on the milk, some farmers now use automatic milking machines to allow cows to decide what suits them.

Experience has shown that when we mess with nature, we often create unexpected problems, e.g. a WHO report in 2011 suggests over-fishing has led to a loss of big fish preying on smaller fish, leading to a marked increase in small fish and jellyfish. Some think this could lead to a possible collapse of the fishing industry by 2050.[92]

Feeding other fish to some farmed fish seems illogical and inefficient, when you consider 5kg of anchovies produces 1kg of salmon. We should also focus on buying quality, including only sustainable fish species.

Issues of human welfare are important in food production, to ensure slaves or bonded labourers, who work long hours and endure poor living conditions, are not used. Whilst there are organisations that monitor working conditions worldwide, problems still exist. A documentary on the tea industry, using hidden cameras, showed untrained workers using pesticides inappropriately that could have an effect on them, as well as the consumer.

A report in 2012 highlighted ongoing child labour and trafficking in Africa, akin to slavery, in the chocolate industry. [www.cnn.com/chocolate]

All this takes us back to asking for evidence of good practice before we buy, as the examples are likely the tip of the iceberg, highlighting a need for more social responsibility to question the morality of activities associated with food production, and a focus on profits, at the expense of welfare, health and safety issues.

As the world's population grows, we need to take a serious look at whether to use water to produce protein by way of livestock or agriculture. Plants can be a source of protein and generally use much less water per unit of production, so does feeding 40% of the world's grain to livestock make sense?

A report from the UK (2012) suggests the amount of food overeaten could feed an extra billion of the world's population. On top of this, wasted food contains about 6% of the United Kingdom's water consumption and New Zealand wastes $750 million worth of food annually. A documentary in 2011 highlighted the huge amount of food that is dumped by supermarkets in the USA, with 'dumpster divers' - salvaging much of it from waste bins, claiming it is fit to eat. [93]

Deficiencies and disease

Now we've considered some general issues about food quality, we can take a closer look at the link between deficiencies and diseases. Just as we appreciate that a sad-looking plant with yellowing leaves needs nutrients to thrive, so too may our bodies, however, the symptoms are usually not so obvious.

A study done at the University of Texas found deceased people had deficiencies of key nutrients including: folic acid, co-enzyme Q10, iodine, magnesium, zinc, chromium, selenium, copper, manganese, vitamins D and C, boron and omega-3 fatty acids. A study at Otago University in New Zealand suggests significant numbers of troops may have died in the First World War due to poor nutrition. Nutritional deficiencies caused by poor lifestyle, environmental factors and some medicines are associated with many diseases.[94]

In *New Nutrition*, Dr Michael Colgan suggests the widespread use of synthetic NPK fertilizer (i.e. nitrogen, phosphate and potassium, whose chemical symbol is K) resulted from a desire to make use of the stockpiles of chemicals remaining after the Second World War.

Dr Colgan stresses that synthetic fertilisers made from fossil fuels upset the balance of nature, when they replace legumes, such as lupins, that return nitrogen from the air to the soil, using energy from the sun, via photosynthesis. He suggests this has led to soil deficiencies and crops more attractive to insect pests and vulnerable to disease. This has resulted in the use of more pesticides, the emergence of industrial agriculture and what he calls 'empty foods' that look all right, but lack the key elements for health, i.e. trace minerals, vitamins and polyphenols that play many roles, including plant preservation and antioxidant activity.

The diagnosis of deficiencies often requires intensive detective work, as some can be extremely subtle. In other circumstances the effect is dramatic, e.g. years ago in New Zealand vast tracts of land were deemed 'useless' for farming, until it was discovered the problem was a soil deficiency of cobalt.

We need to be careful in our research, though. A disease associated with a nutritional abnormality does not automatically prove a cause, e.g. researchers thought that increased homocysteine concentrations caused heart disease. Now, it seems, it is a marker of inflammation, and not the direct cause. Deficiencies may cause slight changes in your general wellbeing, so be careful not to put them down to 'being tired' or 'old age' without expert advice. In some cases, blood tests are available to check for deficiencies.

Sometimes cravings are a sign that your body is telling you there is some sort of imbalance or deficiency. Whilst most people are aware of the importance of iron, folic acid and iodine in pregnancy, there are many nutritional deficiencies linked to diseases, so let's look at a few, to give you a wider perspective.

Iodine deficiency

Here is a summary of iodine deficiency information, taken from the lengthy document on www.health.govt.nz

Iodine is an important constituent of thyroid hormones that maintain the body's metabolic state, normal growth and development. The iodine content of New Zealand soils is low, so locally produced foods may be low in iodine (unless corrected with appropriate fertilization.) Iodine deficiency occurred in New Zealand in the late 1800s and early 1900s, when goitre (neck swelling due to enlarged thyroid gland) was common. To improve the situation table salt was iodised. Recent evidence indicates that the iodine status of New Zealanders is declining again. One way to address this has been to add iodine to commercially prepared bread.

Iodine is essential for normal brain development, and requirements increase during pregnancy and breastfeeding, so it is important that unborn babies and young children have adequate intakes. Whilst a study of breast-fed infants showed iodine levels of less than half that of formula-fed infants, this is not a reason to switch to bottle-feeding, but why the Ministry of Health recommends pregnant and breastfeeding women take a

150microgram iodine tablet daily, available on prescription and subsidised by the government.

Breast milk is associated with many benefits over baby formulae that typically contain high levels of common salt (sodium chloride), which may lead to high blood pressure in later life.

Even with a well-balanced diet, it is difficult to get enough iodine from food alone. Food sources include iodised salt, seafood, milk and eggs. While consumption of iodine supplements and kelp tablets increase intake, take care to avoid an overdose, as the margin between too much and too little is narrow. Also, the iodine content of seaweed and kelp tablets is variable, so consult a health professional.

Iodised salt is a source of iodine, yet the salt may lead to high blood pressure. However, the reputable Cochrane Collaboration Group suggests there is little evidence for this, except when one already has high blood pressure or heart or kidney disease.[95] Whilst salt restriction gives a modest reduction in blood pressure, it may adversely affect cholesterol and adrenaline levels, which could explain an Italian study that suggests too low a salt intake may increase the risk in heart failure patients.

Heart surgeon Dr Oz suggests salt dramatically affects only 10% of the population, with some races more sensitive to it than others. Intake is dependent on physiological demands including sweating and exercise. The Ministry of Health recommends choosing iodised salt when using salt, without increasing overall salt intake.[96]

Chefs often talk about the importance of seasoning food with salt to makes it taste better. Some promote sea salt, which contains valuable minerals, but generally only a minimum of iodine, so iodised sea salt is better. It is also important to note that taste sensation varies amongst individuals, meaning we may not taste salt in food that others do. New Zealanders consume about 9g of salt per day, five times what is recommended. Taste sensations tend to weaken with regular exposure, which may explain why some diners salt their food before tasting it.

To keep your salt intake under control, check food labels and restrict commonly salted foods like salted snacks, soy sauce, smoked food, hard cheeses, processed foods and processed meats. Consider diluting your salt with herbs, e.g. equal parts salt, smoked paprika and cardamom. A study in the USA found 77% of salt intake came from processed food, 12% from natural produce, 5% from cooking and 6% added at the table. Research to make food taste saltier by adding dextran is underway.[97]

Vitamin B12 deficiency

Vitamin B12 is critical for good health, important for nerve and red blood cells, DNA production, and to slow the ageing process. It is noteworthy that the Japanese generally have high B12 blood levels and many live to over one hundred years of age, so that might be a contributing factor.

Symptoms of a deficiency include lack of energy, memory loss, mood changes, numbing and tingling in the feet, depression and dementia. Oral absorption is dependent on the presence of a substance referred to as 'intrinsic factor,' which is reduced by alcohol, diminished acid in the stomach, aspirin and other medicines.[98]

Animal products are good sources of vitamin B12, so vegetarians, especially vegans, usually need to take a supplement. Many New Zealanders over the age of 65 are deficient in vitamin B12 and a study in the USA found 30% of the population deficient, probably due to them eating less meat and more processed food. Lower levels may occur in meat from stock that has been given antibiotics that interfere with the vitamin's production from bacteria in the stomach.[99]

Folic acid deficiency

Folic acid is a member of the B group vitamins, important for good health. Deficiency is widely recognised by health professionals, especially for pregnant mothers where authorities strongly recommend supplementation three months prior to and during pregnancy, to reduce the incidence of *spina bifida*.

The deficiency is so serious that sixty countries have added folic acid to commercial breads, though New Zealand authorities are awaiting more research results before making this decision.

Folic acid derives its name from foliage, giving us a clue to good sources, e.g. green leafy vegetables, such as kale and spinach. Other sources include wholegrain cereals and legumes. A documentary about an eight-year-old boy, who had many operations for complications of his spina bifida, brings home the power of nutrients to prevent diseases that can impact hugely on individuals and society.

Vitamin D deficiency

Vitamin D is important for the correction of DNA errors in our genes and control of calcium in our bodies. Research at the University of Auckland suggests it also plays a major role in a healthy immune system and a number of diseases including: cancers (ironically melanoma), stroke, heart problems, insulin resistance, allergy, osteoporosis, high blood pressure, diabetes, auto-immune diseases, depression, chronic pain, osteoarthritis, muscle weakness and wasting, birth defects, gum disease, multiple sclerosis and Alzheimer's disease.[100] [101]

Reduced sun exposure and use of sunscreens, out of a fear of contracting skin cancer, are major causes of vitamin D deficiency. Michael Holick of the University of Boston suggests 'it is the most common medical condition in the world today' and that some people may need to take vitamin D throughout their lifetime.

The sun and cholesterol combine to provide our body with the best source of vitamin D. Some researchers say not washing for two hours after exposure assists the production of vitamin D.

Whilst we can store vitamin D for 30 to 60 days, deficiency can be a particular problem in winter for those in countries far from the equator (especially beyond 40deg.), or for those of darker skin tones, or who rarely go outside. Food sources include oily fish (cod liver oil, salmon, trout, sardines and kippers), eggs, mushrooms and milk. Vitamin D exists in a number of forms, the best being D3.

Calcium deficiency

Calcium is the most abundant mineral in our bodies with vitamin D important to maintain normal levels. It does this by assisting absorption, decreasing excretion via the kidneys and aiding resorption (re-uptake) from bone, reducing the risk of osteoporosis (weak bones), a condition that affects mainly women over the age of 60 years.[102]

Recent research has linked calcium in supplements to an increased risk of heart attack and strokes. However, the Mayo Clinic says the problem usually occurs when taken without vitamin D and that complementary supplements of magnesium, silicon and boron (in which New Zealand soils are deficient), subject to blood tests.[103] [104]

We absorb about 30% of the calcium in milk and this reduces as we age and in those with low stomach acid levels, which may be a significant issue for anyone taking medicines to reduce acid release in the stomach.[105] Whilst most people think dairy is the main source of calcium, others include kidney beans, tofu, nuts, whole grains, salmon, eggs, broccoli, dairy, seeds, figs, canned sardines (with bones) and green leafy vegetables, such as spinach, kale and kelp.

Excess intake of minerals like sodium, magnesium and phosphate, often used in soft drinks, can interfere with calcium absorption. [http://www.mayoclinic.org/diseases-conditions/heart-attack/expert-answers/calcium-supplements/faq-20058352].

Some people suggest pasteurisation damages some of the enzymes in it. A proportion of the population are lactose-intolerant, leading to bouts of diarrhoea, stomach cramps and flatulence (or wind.) Lactose-free milk is now available.

Homogenisation alters the natural form of milk to allow absorption of the enzyme xanthine oxidase, the effects of which are unclear. In addition, emulsified fats may go directly into the body (bypassing normal digestion), resulting in stomach and immune reaction problems known as 'leaky gut syndrome.'

Whilst most of our milk comes from A1 cows (a mutation going back many years), A2 milk is available, with some suggesting it is better for us, and that goat's milk is even better.

Heart specialist Dr Oz suggests whole milk products are better than low fat varieties because, when you take out the fat, you upset the natural food balance, leaving too high a concentration of sugars that may affect insulin levels.

Selenium deficiency

Whilst more research is required, it seems adequate levels of the mineral selenium have positive effects on prostate problems; lung, bowel and prostate cancer; asthma, the ability to become pregnant, reduction of miscarriages, stroke after-effects, depression and our immune system.

Researchers are now suggesting low blood levels, partly due to low levels of selenium in soil in New Zealand, are a real cause for concern.[106] A good friend, David Walpole has spent years raising awareness of this issue, after discovering problems with livestock, when farming.[107] Farmers in Finland monitor soil levels and apply the mineral as appropriate. In areas of China, where soil levels are low, it is added to table salt.[108]

Some years ago a US company marketed a vitamin and mineral supplement in New Zealand. Because it did not contain selenium, we did not stock it in our pharmacy, and told the company why. To their credit, they eventually added it into their product. At the time of release, a high profile person in New Zealand who probably knew nothing about the selenium issue was endorsing the product. Food sources include meat, fish, eggs and nuts (particularly Brazil nuts).

Food additives

Additives are appearing in more foods today, generally falling into five major groups: sweetening, flavouring (including enhancers like MSG), colouring, emulsifying and preserving. Soy, salt, sugar and thickeners are also more common.

Whilst some play important roles, others, like colouring agents, are more about marketing and may pose health hazards, e.g. in 2012, even though they dispute a colouring additive causes cancer, Coke and Pepsi removed it from their drinks rather than add a cancer warning to their labels to comply with Californian laws.

Earlier we saw the withdrawal of red dye No. 2, associated with cancer, and learned of allergy problems with amaranth. Sometimes additives are illegal, as in the case of sulphite preservative found in fresh red meat in New Zealand in 2013. Sadly, in releasing this story to the media without details of who had done it, the authorities created 'guilt by association'.

Food labels

New Zealand law requires ingredients be listed from the highest to lowest amount, making it easy to see the main ingredients. This can be helpful to detect fake foods, e.g. a can of real blueberry jam will have blueberry near the top of the list, whereas 'blueberry-flavoured' jam will not.

Sometimes misconceptions sway us in the wrong direction, e.g. a chocolate biscuit may be healthier than a savoury cracker laced with TFAs. This shows how important it is to check labels and communicate with manufacturers if unsure. Also, focus on nutrients per 100g, to avoid confusion over portion sizes.

Terms like wholegrain, multigrain and wholewheat can be misleading, if not defined by authorities, or where only a portion in a product allows it to be labelled as such. Beware of misleading marketing, claiming a point of difference by playing on emotions, e.g. terms like 'free range' to describe hens housed in a barn with limited access to the outside world, meaning few actually go there.

A term like 'fat free' often means fat has been replaced by sugar that your body may convert to fat anyway. 'Diet' products contain artificial sweeteners instead of sugar. 'Toasted' often means fried. 'All natural' does not mean much as sugar, fat and oil are all natural. 'No added sugar' products may still contain fruit or milk sugars. 'Light' could mean less fat, less sugar or less salt, but might just refer to taste, colour, density, energy content or potency.

Vague terms such as 'access to pasture' are not easily enforceable; you'd need to consider following the trail of supply right back to the origin. Beware of fancy labelling and packaging to disguise junk food.

The European Union grades food according to traffic light colours, i.e. red indicates high fat levels; orange, moderate levels and green, low levels. This enables shoppers to quickly assess healthy aspects of food, e.g. foods with green indicators are healthier and to be preferred over red. Many doctor groups, including the British Medical Association support the concept and it seems welcomed by consumers.

Despite worries from some in the food industry that foods with 'red' indicators would be shunned,' the British Medical Association and the UK Food Standards Agency say consumers interpret the labels sensibly, realising they can have 'red' foods as an occasional treat and find the labels easier to understand than lists of percentages.[109]

New Zealand uses the Heart Foundation tick system with a recent introduction of the two-tick category.[110]

New Zealand Food Safety Authority (NZFSA) gazetted a new Standard 1.2.7 in January 2013 to ensure food labels making nutritional and health claims provide adequate information for consumers, e.g. reduced fat is less than 25% that in a reference food and low fat is less than 1.5g/ 100ml of liquid or less than 3g/100g of solid. The new standards reduce the risk of misleading and deceptive claims, expand the range of permitted claims and allow industry to innovate to give consumers a wider range of healthy food choices.

Currently meat, fruit and vegetables come with virtually no nutritional information so, hopefully, we will see improvements including; origin, humane treatment and environmental pollution, etc., especially as livestock in New Zealand are now being electronically tagged. Potentially, this will allow buyers to trace the specific source of their meat.

Whilst research suggests people are not always prepared to pay extra for quality, improvements in the availability of reliable information, may make a difference. For more information, go to www.foodstandards.gov.au or www.foodsmart.govt.nz, or the NZFSA (Phone free to 0800-693721.)

Expiry dating of foods in New Zealand involves two systems, i.e. 'best before,' a reflection of quality; and 'use by,' a reflection of safety, which could be dangerous, if ignored. It is important to appreciate an expiry date is based on ideal conditions throughout the supply chain and may be shortened if the recommended storage conditions have not been met. In some instances, authorities may extend an expiry date if storage conditions are better than specified, or tests indicates this is appropriate.

Oestrogens in food

Over the years, there has been a steady rise in the amount of oestrogens, also called phyto (derived from plants)-oestrogens, especially in foods like soy. The world now consumes around 200 million tonnes of soy a year, a significant amount of which is genetically modified.

What amount of oestrogens pose a hazard is not clear, but they are associated with decreased sperm counts. One beer doubles oestrogen levels for about four hours and can be responsible for men developing enlarged breasts. Oestrogens can get into food from packaging and pesticide residues.

Oestrogen-containing foods may also contain phytates, discussed earlier, and enzyme inhibitors (anti-nutrients), the significance of which is unclear. Oestrogens may pose a risk factor for breast cancer, especially for females who menstruated before the age of twelve, used oral contraceptives, had children later in life, bottle-fed their babies, went into menopause after 55 years of age or were prescribed hormone replacement therapy.

Variety and superfoods

Variety is the spice of life and particularly true for nutrition, so aim to eat different foods each day. Not only does variety keep you interested, it increases your chances of getting about 50 'essential' nutrients your body needs from the environment, to limit the risk of deficiencies and associated diseases.

Beware of focusing too much on particular foods to correct nutrients at the expense of 'balanced eating,' where smaller amounts come from a range of foods. An example would be focusing too much on dairy, to build calcium and upsetting the cholesterol balance.

Many phyto-chemicals in our food, essential for good health, are colourful. By thinking about eating foods according to the colours of a rainbow, you have a simple way to get a good mix of what are often referred to as superfoods. The mnemonic **'Roy G. Biv'** will help you to remember the colours: red, orange, yellow (and white), green, blue, indigo and violet.

Eating about 600g of colourful fruits and vegetables per day is associated with reduced susceptibility to disease, but note that green chlorophyll can mask colourful nutrients in plants.

Superfoods include - spirulina, avocado, bee pollen, oysters, royal jelly, berries (especially blueberries, lingonberries, and strawberries), cinnamon (not cheap imitations), citrus, green (higher levels) and black tea, green leafy vegetables, salmon, chia seeds, walnuts, sweet potato, resveratrol (grape seed and skin), almonds, tomatoes, beetroot, rolled oats, beans, kiwifruit, cruciferous vegetables (broccoli, cabbage and Brussels sprouts), garlic, onions and dark chocolate, containing 70% cocoa (maximum of 25g per day).

Varieties of produce are being developed with improved nutritional value, e.g. Monty's surprise apple, claimed to have extra cancer fighting properties.

To help select superfoods, look for the ORAC score (oxygen radical absorbance capacity), a method of measuring the antioxidant capacity of foods and supplements, developed by scientists at the National Institutes of Health in the USA. Whilst the exact relationship between the ORAC value of a food and health benefits are not clear, foods that score higher on the scale neutralise free radicals more effectively.

Beware of products marketed as superfoods that are overpriced and offer little or no benefit over common fruits and vegetables. For example, a study reported in the Australian *Choice* magazine looked at nine 'superfood juices' and found antioxidant activity of a 30ml serving was less than a Red Delicious apple, a reminder of the importance of doing your own research.

CHAPTER 13

What is a Healthy Lifestyle?

Energy and exercise

The old 'calories in, calories out' model has fallen out of favour, though many still use it as a rough guide. You cannot exercise off calories, and equate this to what you have eaten, as it depends whether the calories came from real or processed food, and what nutrients were present at the time. Health and well-being guru Chris Kresser discusses this further at www.chriskresser.com.

Two units of energy are used around the world, i.e. calories (cal) and kilojoules (kJ). A calorie (cal/kcal) equals 4.184kJ, often rounded to 4 for convenience of calculation. For nutrition, the abbreviations 'cal' and 'kcal' are synonymous. This came about because the unit used in nutrition is 1000 times greater than that used in scientific work.

An average adult female requires about 8,370 kJ (2,000cal) and the average adult male about 10,600 kJ (2,500cal) per day. Carbohydrates and protein provide 17kJ (4cal)/g; alcohol 30 kJ (7cal)/g and fats and oils 38 kJ (9cal)/g.

Energy, calories or kilojoules are different terms for the same thing. The amount of energy you need depends on a number of factors including height, age, weight, muscle mass, gender, physical activity, climate and whether you want to maintain, lose or gain weight. Over half of the energy you use powers your organs and bodily functions such as heart pumping, digestion and brain activity.

Famous nutritionist, Michael Colgan said, "If you don't have time for exercise, you leave time for disease." The motto 'use it or lose it' also provides a good message, including the value of weight-bearing exercise to maintain strong muscles and bones.

The World Health Organisation recommends one hour of moderate activity, every day to improve health, increase metabolism and prevent obesity. You do not have to be active within that one block of time, as a few minutes here and there all add up.

Many factors determine how much energy you use exercising, including height, weight, metabolic rate, so you will need to consult websites, etc., to calculate specifics. As a guide, if you walk slowly at 2km/hour, your body burns about 2cal (8.4 kJ) a minute. Double this and you are reaching moderate physical activity where you start to experience health benefits, even though you may not lose weight. Think carefully about the energy you burn exercising, so as not to counteract it with too much food or energy drinks. Water is preferable to sports drinks for average exercise sessions under one hour. Seek professional advice for endurance exercise.

High intensity interval training (HIIT) combining short bursts of high intensity exercise followed by low intensity recovery periods has gained interest in recent times. An example includes that of Tony Horton, featured on the Dr Oz show. His program consists of ten minutes of serious activity for a minimum of five days a week. He stresses it is important to exercise for the right reasons and not be too hard on yourself as this makes success harder to achieve.

Introduce fitness to children early, but avoid weights for those under eight years of age. Combine a healthy, balanced diet with your exercise.[111] Interestingly, Massey School of Sports Medicine in New Zealand has done a small study and found benefits in blueberries for muscle recovery.

Be sure to warm up before exercise, especially for stressful activities, then warm down and stretch at the end. If you are not involved in specific activities, aim for 10,000 steps a day to maintain weight and 15,000 steps to lose weight, confirmed with a pedometer for good measure.

Whilst exercise should involve the whole body, the important thing is that you do something and build up slowly to a point where it becomes a habit and you hardly notice. Some professionals have recommended exercising at your optimal heart rate, but this is now questioned by some.[112]

It is important to remember that activities like mowing the lawn, housework, raking leaves and a game of sport are all forms of exercise. Consider also options such as taking the stairs instead of the lift, parking the car further away from your destination and walking, or even leaving it at home and walking or cycling. In fact, we should consider replacing the word 'exercise' with something like 'activity' to get away from negative associations, e.g. going to a gym, strenuous exercise and sweaty bodies.

If you plan to increase you activity, arrange for a medical check first to ensure you are not suffering from undetected conditions like high blood pressure that may pose a risk. Also, be aware that medicine to control blood pressure may be less effective when exercising.

Ask your gym instructor for details of their qualifications to reduce the chances of injury from being taught poor techniques, etc. Some gyms hold sessions specifically for the very overweight in rooms without mirrors or public windows to avoid the embarrassment of working out alongside healthy athletes with impressive bodies, etc.

Do not overdo exercise, as researchers at the Mayo Clinic in the USA (2012) have found more than one hour of intense aerobic exercise per day may increase the risk of premature death from heart problems. [www.mayoclinic.org]

Visit http://www.mayoclinic.org/healthy-living/fitness/in-depth/fitness/art-20048269 for advice on how to start a daily exercise program and do not forget to exercise your brain also with reading, puzzles, brain-gym exercises, etc.

Water

Water hydrates and provides a medium for biological functions and for flushing toxins from your body. Whilst the consensus seems to be we need about 30ml of water per kg per day, the Cochrane group suggests there is little evidence this is true (which does not mean it is untrue).[113] Some people flavour drinking water with herbs, etc., and advocate drinking about 500ml first thing each morning.[114] A glass of water, half an hour before meals, may reduce appetite.

As we age our thirst reflex tends to weaken, so we may not feel thirsty until dehydrated (loss of 1% bodyweight), hence drink regularly to avoid the consequences, e.g. muscle cramps, constipation, nervous system effects and kidney stones. A crude check for dehydration is to pinch the skin on the back of the hand and see how quickly it returns to normal. Anything that provides a reminder to drink water is helpful, including fridges with chilled water dispensers on the front and dispensers in waiting rooms and workplaces.

Caffeine in tea, coffee, chocolate and cola drinks has a diuretic effect (i.e. it increases urine output), especially if you are not that active, or increase your dose of caffeine by having extra-strong drinks. Take note of the effect on your body and drink extra water to correct any imbalance.[115]

Quality water is critical for health and survival. However, chlorine in water supplies guards us from infection, though some recommend removing it before drinking. Normal filtration removes solid material and bacteria only if the filter is extremely fine. To get rid of a dissolved chemical such as chlorine, we need to use distillation, or filters containing activated charcoal to adsorb (chemically bind) it. [www.nsf.org]

The Ministry of Health recommends running the tap for a few seconds in the morning, before drinking to limit exposure to a build-up of copper, etc., overnight. For the same reason, do not drink water from the hot water tap from a copper storage tank.

Overseas studies have found town water supplies contaminated with arsenic, lead, chromium-6, radon, asbestos, microbes, perchlorate, herbicides, pesticides and medicines, none of which are good for your health. In 2013, some rural water supplies in New Zealand were found to contain high levels of nitrates that could be dangerous for pregnant women and bottle-fed babies (resulting in the 'blue baby syndrome.') If in any doubt about the quality of your water, ask to see test results, rather than just taking someone's word for it.

More people are buying water in plastic bottles these days. If you do, be sure to ask those good probing questions, e.g. does it contain chlorine, how are containers recycled, where does the water come from, how safe are the plastics, are the bottles sealed in the factory to eliminate tampering etc., and do I really need to get it this way?

Food portions

The Ministry of Health (NZ) recommends the following each day:

	SERVINGS
Vegetables	3
Fruit	2
Wholegrain bread/cereal/rice and pasta	6
Milk/cheese/yoghurt and ice cream	2
Lean meat/poultry/seafood	1
Eggs/nuts/seeds/ legumes	1

Serving size

Easy guides to the food quantities recommended as a single serving include the amount fitting on the palm of your hand or on common household objects, as follows:

- A deck of cards or a flat hand for a serving of meat.
- 2 to 3 CDs is about 60-80g of cheese.
- A slice of bread.
- A fist or tennis ball for a serving of carbs, e.g. cereal, rice or pasta.
- 1 to 2 tablespoonful of fats/oils per day.[116]

The concept of the 'food pyramid' has long been popular, ideally shown upside down so the main foods get appropriate attention. Alternatively, a diagrammatical plate of food, modified from www.choosemyplate.gov (U.S Department of Agriculture), gives you an idea of the balance of foods to eat at most meals, as follows:

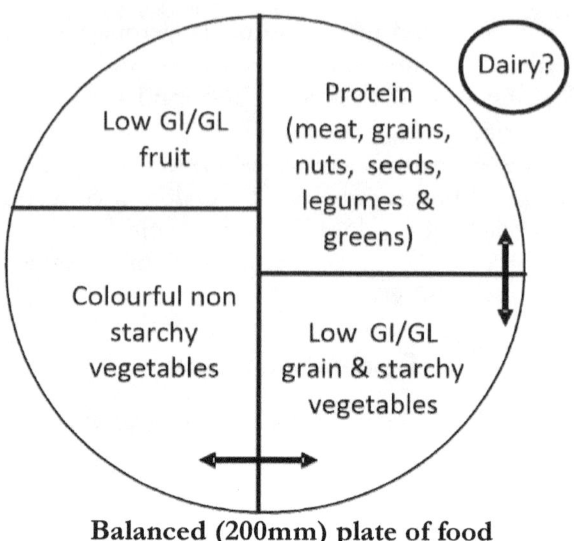

Balanced (200mm) plate of food

The arrows indicate variations according to your metabolic type, as discussed. The protein portion in the diagram helps to make a move toward a more plant-based diet. Dairy is not essential. Focusing on a balanced plate of food at most meals avoids having to think of details.

Over the years, we have seen a move towards super-sizing all kinds of objects, e.g. houses, cars, boats and fast food combos. This has included larger dinner plates where a 200mm (8 inch) diameter plate typically holds about 800cal (3,360kJ) and a 300mm (12 inch) diameter plate holds twice as much, equalling nearly a whole day's calorie intake at a single meal. Reserve those extra-large plates for skeet shooting and remember what actually goes on your plate is what matters most.[117]

Weight issues

As we age, our metabolism slows, along with our level of activity, meaning we need less food. Unless we adjust for this, we will gain weight. Today many people are overfed and overweight, yet under-nourished, through excess consumption of poor quality food. Get out some photos of yourself in earlier times - they could be the wake-up call you need.

Diabesity by Dr Francine Kaufman demonstrates the links between diabetes and obesity. She estimates there are two billion severely overweight (obese) people in the world, with hospitals under pressure to provide special facilities for them.

Because a person could have high levels of fat in their body yet not appear overweight, certain body-fat measurements are important. The average male body contains 15% to 20% fat (over 25% is high) and the average female body contains 20% to 27% fat (over 35% is high.)

Fat tests include the Body Mass Index (BMI), calculated by dividing a person's weight (kg) by the square of their height, in metres. Refer to the BMI table below to check how you rate, bearing in mind that research in 2012 suggests this tool may underestimate how much fat you are carrying.

Sex	Desirable BMI	Overweight BMI	Obese BMI
Female	18.7 - 23.5	23.6 - 28.2	>28.2
Male	20.5 - 25.0	25.0 - 30.0	>30.0

Another fat test is the ratio of waist to hip measurements where women above 0.85 and men above 0.9 are high.[118] Portable testing machines are also available.

Dr G. Gaesser (PhD in exercise physiology) suggests that body weight may not be as significant an issue as most think. He says, "You can be fit, yet fat, and that we need to focus more on fitness and reduce what some people call 'yo-yo' dieting, i.e. losing and gaining weight on a cyclical basis. What we eat and how much we exercise causes blood vessel plaque, not obesity."

He believes it is possible to reduce risk factors, without losing weight, and suggests population information about obesity may be misleading, because much relies on self-reporting surveys. Thin people have heart attacks, too, and fitness may be easier than losing weight. However, do not get smug about this, as being overweight is a risk factor for a number of diseases.

The ability to put on weight when food was plentiful and get by in times of famine was a key survival trait in prehistoric times. Today modern man has access to a wide variety of quality foods from around the world, throughout the year, giving rise to a diet that has changed more in the last fifty years than the previous 1,000 years, with the human body struggling to adapt. With food so readily available, many people are storing fat for a famine that will never come.

Recent research shows disruption of hormones can play an important part in eating habits, e.g. ghrelin makes us hungry, with levels in some who are overweight remaining higher than normal, so they are continually hungry. During eating, levels of the hormone leptin rise to lower motivation to eat. Again, in the overweight, the rise may be less than normal. Dr T. Spector at King's College, London, is currently studying groups of twins that have contrasting weights, to find some answers.

Ongoing research, highlighted by G. Weston, surgeon and author, and Dr C Le Roux of the Imperial College, London has found gastric bypass operations not only shrink the size of the stomach (and the amount of food absorbed), but somehow affects the brain (as recorded through MRI scans), to improve eating habits.

Research reported in *The New England Journal of Medicine* in 2011 confirms that if we significantly cut back on food, the body switches into preservation mode, and stores as much energy as possible, as fat. Ghrelin levels spike and metabolism drops after the cut, so most dieters regain the weight they have lost.

Researchers at Melbourne University (Proietto *et al*) have even detected what they call the 'post-diet syndrome' whereby, a full year after significant weight loss, patients remained in a 'biologically altered state' with their bodies acting as if they were starving, with high levels of ghrelin and low levels of leptin. They also found the human body continues fighting against weight loss for a long time, with muscles becoming more efficient and able to burn 25% less calories doing the same amount of work.

There may even be a link between obesity and microbes in the stomach, where certain bacteria cause release of nutrients in food that would have remained undigested in lean people.

Dr N. Barnard, a USA nutritionist, believes overeating is an addiction to salty, sweet and fatty foods that trigger release of dopamine in the brain to make us feel good. Some people have fewer dopamine receptors, so eat more to get that same feeling.

Research now suggests a link between obesity and ADHD disease, possibly due to adult sufferers having less ability to plan healthy meals.

As these ideas gain acceptance, we will see changes in attitudes from unfortunate situations where some health professionals will not deal with overweight patients, because they see them as lazy gluttons who cannot help themselves. Clearly, it is much more complicated than this.

I trust your mind is now open to the fact that weight control is not as simple as many believe, but please do not use this as an excuse to do nothing. There is no magic bullet, but admittedly we can be tempted into thinking there is, when research suggests low levels of a type of hormone called adiponectin are associated with being overweight [www.realdose.com], and magnesium in foods like pumpkin seeds corrects this. The danger is when people grasp at 'a magic bullet' like this, but ignore other important aspects of their health in the process.

The self-image you have about your weight is important. Visualise yourself with your ideal body weight and repeat this until it becomes a habit. Beware of your sub-conscious sabotaging your efforts, which may require treatment like neuro-linguistic programming (NLP). Aim to eliminate emotional eating, where food is used to numb low self-esteem, inactivity and stress, and remember weight loss is all about lifestyle change.

Go to www.betterhealthforyou.co.nz and register to receive a software program that shows what nutrients you are getting from your food, to get you started.

Aided by your mentor, be realistic and think about who you are, what you want and why you want it. Ask yourself, why am I overweight? Why do I want to lose weight? Why have I been unable to maintain weight loss in the past?

Healthy food is not only nutritious and filling; often it requires extra chewing that helps to avoid overeating. This is because there is a time delay of about fifteen minutes from when you eat food to when your brain registers what you have eaten. Eat your food slowly and take breaks between courses. Not only will this aid your digestive enzymes, it also makes it easier to know when you've eaten enough.

Beware of old habits like eating everything on your plate, influenced by times of food shortages. Know the importance of stopping when you're satiated. Turntables are one way of letting people select small portions at a time. Be careful, though: research suggests some people eat up to 25% more than they need, if food is there in front of them.

Simpson and Raubenheimer of *The Nature of Nutrition* suggest higher costs means more people are eating less animal protein and over-eating fats and carbohydrates in the process. Moreover, not all calories are created equal, so after eating the same calories of nuts or French fries, you will likely eat more food at your next meal after the fries, as the nuts take longer to digest and the fries stimulate insulin release, making you feel hungrier earlier.

This underlies growing evidence that being overweight has much to do with consumption of highly processed, high GI/GL man-made carbohydrates, leading to insulin resistance and increased conversion of carbohydrates to fat.[119] Fat around the stomach associates with Syndrome X; Type 2 diabetes; cancer; heart disease and high cortisol levels and stress - that leads to a craving for carbohydrates, high blood sugars, reduced fat metabolism and the breakdown of muscle.

Focus on low GI/GL foods. Eat anti-inflammatory foods like whole grains, olive and fish oils with varied pace exercise, done at high intensity for short periods. Fat on thighs, arms and buttocks is better than having it around the stomach area, but is harder to reduce.

If you significantly reduce food intake, glycogen converts to glucose for energy and releases roughly 2kg of water (attached to the glycogen.) So most of the initial weight loss is water. Weight regain may occur, because the body tends to store a larger amount of glycogen and water. This illusion of easy weight loss, followed by a demoralising weight gain, highlights the importance of not relying on scales, but initially concentrating on increased activity and healthy eating.[120]

Market surveys suggest most of us think in terms of what we eat, not how much we eat, so we start with swapping to healthier foods without thinking about portion sizes. Obsessing on measurements may lead to disappointment and cause some people to give up.[121] Because muscle is denser than fat, it's possible to gain weight as you increase activity and replace fat with muscles, that burn energy, which is good.

Children who eat at least three meals a week with their family at the dining table are more likely to eat healthily, maintain an ideal bodyweight and display other health benefits.[122] A UK study found 40% of pregnant women had an inadequate diet, with some researchers believing an overweight mother could be the cause of an overweight child.[123] Fat cells developed in childhood and teenage years remain, seeking fat, which explains why there is a tendency for overweight children to be overweight adults. In addition, an overweight person is much more likely to have an overweight spouse.[124]

Nudge factors are environmental factors such as how food is displayed that affect behaviour. In one study, researchers found positive effects on the type and amount of food selected from a breakfast buffet, when healthy food dominated the display, and mirrors gave diners a reminder of their body shape.

Many a time in the pharmacy I have listened to customers complaining about painful knees and hips and long waiting lists for surgery. Often I was tempted to suggest they take a good look in the mirror and consider how much their being overweight contributed to the problem.

I mentioned this to a doctor friend who said, "You couldn't do that." Maybe political correctness holds us back from saying things that are in a patient's best interest. Interestingly, research suggests that if you are obese, losing 5kg could reduce your risk of developing arthritis by 50%.[125]

Anyone with fewer taste buds (shown by low sensitivity to hot chilli peppers) tends to eat more to stimulate them. Keep your tongue sensitive by replacing some fats with herbs.

Some people overeat when the food is bland, so tastier food could lower consumption.[126] Childhood ear infections can damage taste nerves that may lead to overeating.

Enjoy three meals a day, selecting from dishes that encourage you to eat plant foods and fish, with little or no deep-fried food.

Eat fewer foods high in fat, added sugars, preservatives and salt, e.g. cakes, cookies, ice cream, sweets, sweetened drinks, pizza, sausages, bacon and hot dogs.

Use only small amounts of fats and oils, sugar and salt when cooking and preparing meals, snacks or drinks. Choose ready-prepared foods low in these ingredients.

Other key points:

You should be hungry before you eat.	If it is not natural, do not eat it.
Avoid crash diets as your body can only lose about 1.5kg fat per week.	A tightening waistband may be a warning sign for action.
Beware of oversized 'man-size' portions and the number of portions per pack.	Consult a health professional before undergoing a weight-loss program.
Breakfast like a king, lunch like a prince and dine like a pauper.	Thinner people taste fat before others, so therefore eat less of it. (Deakin University, Australia)
Do not skip meals regularly as you are likely to make up for it later.	Lack of sleep leads to low metabolism and increased appetite.
Link food to your body make-up or metabolic type, e.g. a muscular person may need more protein.	Some bodies seem programmed for a particular weight, but that setting can be changed. [127] [128]
Beware of overeating at buffets.	Some medicines cause weight gain.
Deficiencies of trace minerals like manganese and chromium may cause over eating.	Hollywood stars have popularised the gluten-free diet that was devised for those diagnosed with coeliac disease.
Significantly cutting back on food makes us hungry, which can lead to reducing activity to compensate.	It might be that vegetarians who are overweight think they can eat more treats because they are on 'a healthy diet.'

Modern day diets

According to many experts, the Western diet, focused on refined, fatty, salty and poor nutrition foods, is associated with many serious health issues including diabetes, obesity, cancer and heart disease and is an example of what eating should not be. Noticeable drops in health occur when there's a change from traditional healthy diets to this.

Now let us see what we can learn from some of the multitude of diets (eating plans) on the market. Most are devised to help with weight loss; some are intended to treat specific conditions through clinical nutrition. Remember, you are unique. Go for ideas that could help you achieve your goals.

Dr D. Ornish of the Preventative Medicine Research Institute promotes a low fat, plant-based wholefood diet combined with daily half-hour walks, stretching and relaxation through yoga, meditation, group sessions for emotional support and no smoking. For this he claims a 75% drop in artery clogging.

Dr Oz's approach is to increase metabolism. Start by knowing your basal metabolic rate (BMR), based on age, activity, height and weight. Set goals, make minimal cuts in carbohydrate intake, add more protein to reduce hunger, avoid being hungry by eating healthy snacks, e.g. nuts or dried fruit between meals up to 8pm.

Other tips: three iced drinks a day helps the body use more energy in warming them. Take zinc, because leptin that reduces appetite depends on this mineral. Exercise in bursts to wake up the muscles. Metabolic boosters such as white bean extract, L-Arginine and pickled peppers may help. Chris Powell, a guest on his show, promotes alternate high and low carbohydrate days. Tim Ferris, also a guest, suggests a 3-minute cold shower in the morning to activate brown fat, which burns calories.

The Diogenes (**Di**et, **O**besity, **Genes**) Group Study compared high and low protein and low GI/GL diets and concluded high protein, low fat, low GI/GL diets work best. [129] In *Prevent and Reverse Heart Disease* Caldwell and Esselstyn recommend wholegrain cereals, breads and pastas; fruits and vegetables, with little or no oil, meat or dairy products.[130]

The '**DASH**' diet - **D**ietary **a**pproach to **s**top **h**ypertension (high blood pressure) recommends low fat and salt, ten servings of fruit and vegetables per day, three servings of low fat dairy, wholegrains, poultry, fish, a little red meat and few sugary foods.[131]

The Macrobiotic Diet avoids processed foods in favour of natural, organic food traditionally cooked. Microwaving is prohibited and slow eating and thorough chewing advised.

The Atkins Diet discusses the fact that too many highly processed carbs leads to insulin resistance with conversion to fat and that the body burns fat when carbs are replaced with fat and protein, ideally for a short time.[132]

The Alkalinising Diet - In 1931 Nobel Prize winner Dr Otto Warburg came up with the idea that weakened cell respiration (due to a lack of oxygen at the cellular level) results in fermentation. The lactic acid produced lowers cell pH and destroys the ability of DNA and RNA to control division, leading to cancer.

106

Focus on relaxation and alkaline foods like dark leafy greens, most fruit (including citrus) and nuts rather than foods that produce acidic cell conditions such as phosphate in soft drinks, excess sugar, refined grains, saccharin and aspartame. R. Young in *The pH Miracles* advances the idea of testing your saliva pH, where the ideal is 6.8 to 7. *The Healthy Food Guide* says, "Eating more fruit and vegetables increases the intake of vitamins, antioxidants, fibre and increases the alkaline-forming balance in your diet."

You can also live and eat according to your Blood Type Diet.[133] *The Seventeen-Day Diet,* devised by Dr Mike Moreno claims to reset the body's weight-control hormones.[134] The Change One diet advises one change at a time with recipes.[135] The Coronary Health Improvement Program (CHIP) is a vegetarian diet.

An Australian College of Nutritional and Environmental Medicine (ACNEM) paper refers to a 'Low Stress' Diet that is gluten and dairy-free, contains no caffeine or alcohol, and is supplemented with multivitamins, essential fatty acids from fish oil, good bacteria (probiotics) and potent antioxidants.

The Pritikin Diet recommends unprocessed foods like fruits, vegetables, legumes, wholegrains such as brown rice, starchy vegetables, lean meat and seafood, with an emphasis on at least thirty minutes of aerobic exercise such as brisk walking and weight training two to three times weekly, with daily stretching.

Don Tolman suggests that shape gives a clue to the benefits of specific foods for parts of the body, e.g. a cross-section of a carrot resembles the retina of the eye; a celery stalk looks like a long bone and a shelled walnut looks like the brain.[136]

The Cronies Diet (Calorie restriction and optimal nutrition) focuses on low calorie, nutrient-dense, high protein food, (i.e. 10% to 30% calories below normal) with an emphasis on thorough chewing. It claims the diet results in lower blood pressure, improved cholesterol and younger hearts compared to the average USA citizen. Proponents claim it adds up to eight years to a lifespan, through slowed shortening of telomeres in DNA, associated with the ageing process.[137] Along these lines, more attention is focusing on fasting, e.g. alternate days of normal and limited eating. Research is ongoing.

The Food Hospital in the UK, staffed by a surgeon, doctor and dietician, is an example of clinical nutrition in action. These professionals have developed a range of eating plans to treat specific conditions, e.g. an anti-inflammatory plan for psoriasis, low carbohydrate plan for ankylosing spondylitis, an antioxidant plan for acid reflux caused by stress, and a low carb, low GI/GL plan for fatty liver.[138]

The Gerson Diet is natural treatment, developed by Dr M. Gerson in the 1920s, using organic foods, juicing, coffee enemas, detoxification and natural supplements to activate the body's ability to heal itself.[139] A typical juice consists of 3 to 4 carrots, one apple, half a beetroot and a small piece of ginger and possibly a citrus fruit and/or a kiwifruit, to be drunk up to ten times a day. Juicing, that removes most fibre and concentrates nutrition, requires less energy for absorption, so is ideal for seriously ill patients.

The popularity and validity of some weight loss diets (not detailed here) may be exaggerated and expensive or based on false assumptions, e.g. that there was only one caveman/hunter-gather (Paleo) diet.

Buying food

When buying food it is important to develop strategies to get health and value for money. Consider issues such how busy the store is, which reflects stock turnover; cleanliness and customer service, the look and feel of fresh and packaged foods; lighting and temperature control.

Beware of poor impulse buys through powerful marketing tools, e.g. specials, colourful signs, endorsements, strategic shelf positioning and sampling promotions. Do your homework.

Quality food may appear to cost extra, so keep things in perspective by comparing products after the waste is removed, e.g. salmon fillets versus a whole chicken. Beware of specials that are not 'value for money,' e.g. a large bottle of soft drink provides many cheap, but poor quality calories. Layouts tend to be standardised with nutritionists suggesting we limit time in the central aisles that mostly contain highly processed foods, and spend most time in the produce areas on the outside.

One only has to observe a few supermarket trolley loads of food to realise that some people need help with the choices they make. To address this the New Zealand Heart Foundation arranged a dietician to take customers on a 'free tour' of a supermarket to get tips about healthy buying, yet I was the only person who turned up. One especially notable point during our stroll around the aisles was an extra-large display of cheap, white sliced bread, reflecting high sales of this product over the wholegrain varieties that were only a dollar more expensive.

Considering the importance of food, I see a real opportunity for food stores to differentiate themselves from the competition. Some ways this could happen include:

- Independent nutrition experts on hand.
- Displays to help the public understand true (nutritional) quality, the source and value for money, including additive codes used on labels.

- Cost per 100g information on shelves to make price comparisons easier.
- Full and transparent information based on statistically reliable data about the nutrient content, growing methods, amount of water used, etc., for those intent on healthy living and sustainability.
- With many of us so busy these days, shopping online (with delivery) is gaining in popularity. Time saved could be devoted to making healthier choices, especially if nutritional information is available on the website, and repeat orders are easy to do.

Not long after buying our pharmacy, the benefits of cranberries to treat urinary tract infections was recognised. Talking to patients, I discovered doctors were telling them to buy the juice from supermarkets. As we had high-quality, high-potency cranberry capsules for sale, I decided to check out the quality of the juice by writing to a major supplier. I got the curt reply, "The amount of cranberry in our product is commercially sensitive and cannot be released." This suggested they had something to hide. What a shame doctors did not discuss the issue with me beforehand.

Some years ago, my wife and I hosted a dinner party at which we served gelato ice cream. One of our guests noted it was past the expiry date, much to our horror. We had bought it the day before, so returned it to the supermarket, where they gave us a refund. I was there two weeks later and decided to check the expiry of their gelato. To my amazement, the expired stock was still in the freezer.

As the manager kept blaming the supplier, I lodged a complaint with the local health authorities. With modern technology and good stock rotation, this sort of problem should not happen, but it is a reminder to check expiry dates.

Fast foods

Today fast food has become synonymous with pre-cooked, 'energy-dense' food, preying on a human attraction to fat, salt and sugar. The changes have meant less valuable meat stock often end up as foods like burgers to the point we are likely to forget they come from animals. In the process, food technologists are creating a vast array of artificial 'Frankenstein foods,' made from synthetic ingredients unknown to home cooks.

In 2012 a news story featured a woman who spent an entire day preparing and photographing a burger for marketing purposes. The actual product did not look as good as the photograph, yet the New Zealand Commerce Commission ruled this was acceptable, because it had the same ingredients.

Fast food is often about fast service, fast eating; fast rises in blood sugar and a fast return to hunger. Convenience is killing us through the tendency to grab poor quality fast food as an alternative to preparing quality meals at home. Some believe it is linked to the epidemic of diabetes and obesity in India.

Experts suggest unhealthy lifestyles account for two out of five deaths, with fast food making a significant contribution to this shocking statistic, bringing into question the morality of fast food advertisements on uniforms of champion sportsmen (who probably never eat the products) and venues.

New Zealanders spend $1.5 billion each year on fast food and devour 22 litres of ice cream and drink 75 litres of soft drink per person, per year.[140] Around the world many millions of servings of soft drink are consumed every day, much of which contains fructose from sugar or corn syrup and associated with health hazards.

Rumours continue to circulate about the safety of aspartame yet authorities say it is safe at normal levels. However it should not be consumed by people with a disease called Phenylketonuria (PKU).

If we look back through history, roadside stalls, selling a wide variety of foods, were part of the lifestyle. Whilst most people class fast foods as junk food, this is not always the case, e.g. the man who lived on Subway fast food for two years, without any weight gain. In another example, chef Michael Van de Elzen from Auckland has taken to the road in his 'food truck' to promote ways to eat healthier fast food, e.g. baking chips, putting vegetables in meat patties and using wholesome ingredients, instead of those which are highly refined.[141]

A key is to look at the big picture. For example, when reviewing potato chips, a New Zealand survey found some companies used sodium hydroxide to peel potatoes, the average fat content was 11% and the quality and temperature of the oil were important issues to consider. With the trend to using more heat-stable saturated oils like palm oil, more research is required to assess its safety.

Schools are very expensive institutions and we know healthy eating is essential for good brain function and learning. For example, too many carbohydrates for lunch, without adequate protein, may reduce attention spans in the afternoon. Schools provide an ideal opportunity to focus attention on 'quality' food, including projects to monitor consumption and weight, not to mention the flow-on effect into homes.

Maybe we also need widespread adoption of a general term to describe food that is healthy, but quick and easy to prepare, e.g. 'convenience' food. Check for nutritional content of fast food on brochures and websites in order to make wise choices and look for healthy alternatives e.g. the

Wholefoods Market chain of stores focuses on healthy food and provides an area where customers can sit and eat their purchases.

Moderation and food classification

When I was a child, a wonderful teacher put a lot of emphasis on the idea of moderation (temperance) in all things. He stressed how people get into trouble eating, working, exercising, sleeping and drinking alcohol, etc., in excess. Just like our pharmacy patients who developed gout from eating too many beans from their summer garden.

You might be surprised to learn some foods generally considered healthy are on a list of 'not needed' foods for the overweight, published in the *New Zealand Journal of Medicine* in February 2012. The long list includes honey, muesli bars and fruit juice and soon became a 'hot topic' for talkback hosts and the media alike.

Ironically, some members of the public took umbrage that academics could tell them what they should or should not eat. As I listened to the debate, I wondered how many complainants would be prepared to pay for ill health resulting from their poor lifestyle decisions. Whilst the report was useful to get people talking, it tended to demonise fats, and we know not all are bad.

It listed alternatives like processed meats, which, as we have seen, are not to be encouraged. As we saw with the 'Food Truck chef,' it is not easy to categorise foods as good or bad, e.g. not all pies are unhealthy. Much depends on the context in which foods are consumed, e.g. serving deep-fried, high GI/GL potato chips to customer in bars may not be ideal, but is likely to keep blood alcohol levels down and may reduce the chances of a crash, driving home.

Now think about your eating habits, what you would like to change, and how. For instance, my wife and I have a pact to restrict junk food in the house, so as not to be tempted. What food would you have difficulty in giving up, but know you should, especially if you have a weight problem? Consider foods like soft drinks, potato chips, fried foods, white bread, white flour, sugar, regular pasta, high fat products and foods containing artificial colourings, preservatives and flavourings.

In some cases, your craving may be so strong, elimination may not be appropriate, so a reduction might be a better way to go initially. Think about hiding gadgets like the deep fryer and ice cream maker, or focus on using them less often, or to make healthier foods like fruit gelato and wholegrain bread.

Do not be too tough on yourself. Take small steps at a time, replacing 'bad' foods with 'good.' What you eat most of the time is what really matters. Allow yourself occasional treats, e.g. have one day of the week when rules are somewhat relaxed, to make it easier to achieve your goals.

Cravings can be associated with an addiction to some carbohydrates as suggested by Dr Atkins, and studied by Dr Mike Dow and reported in *Diet Rehab* where he talks about addiction to bad foods that can make us feel good by raising the levels of dopamine. Because the effect does not last long, this soon leads to a craving for more. Dr Dow's approach is to focus on gradually replacing 'bad' foods with what he calls 'booster foods' over a 4-week period. He groups his booster foods (all low GI/GL) into certain grains, protein, dairy, fruit and vegetables.[142]

Vitamin and mineral supplements

Many people die or are disabled prematurely from preventable diseases, many of which are linked to nutrition. Vitamins and minerals play crucial roles in the body, transforming food into energy, growth, digestion, elimination, wound healing and resistance to disease. By now you will have an appreciation of how difficult it is to get all the nutrients your body needs from your food, and that even medicines can disrupt this.

It is best to get the majority of your nutrition from good quality food, as poorly formulated supplements may provide nutrients, without the co-factors necessary to be safe and effective. For example, too much vitamin B6 on its own may be harmful, but the foods that contain it, such as avocados, bananas, dried beans and whole grains, also provide nutrients that work with it. The answer might be an alteration in what you eat, how you prepare it, or taking a quality vitamin and mineral supplement with appropriate testing, guidance and knowledge.

I stress the testing, as we have a long way to go before vitamins and minerals levels are routinely measured and monitored. Let us now look at reasons why you might consider taking a vitamin and mineral supplement as a form of insurance.

Whilst some experts say a healthy diet is all you need, *The Journal of the American Medical Association* recommends them, saying, 'most people do not consume an optimal amount of vitamins and minerals by diet alone.'[143] On the other hand, health authorities in the UK caution against widespread use of vitamin and mineral products, as research suggests beta-carotene (natural vitamin A) in them may increase lung cancer in smokers, so maybe they should simply avoid this vitamin.

An increase in dietary intake of antioxidant vitamins has encouraging prospects for heart disease prevention.[144] One study found breast cancer risk most pronounced among women below the median daily consumption of fruits and vegetables.[145] Many nutrients assist eye health including lutein, zeaxanthin, vitamins A, E and C, zinc and selenium reduce the risk of cataract and macular degeneration.[146] [147] [148]

The B group vitamins, zinc and vitamin E play key roles for energy. In today's busy stressful world, many people need extra B group vitamins, especially those who consume above average amounts of alcohol and have poor eating habits.[149]

Many situations pose special risks for deficiencies already discussed, e.g. pregnancy and iron, folic acid and iodine. Others include pollution, living alone, poor appetite, anorexia, bulimia, oral contraceptives, bio-individuality, athletes, premenstrual tension, food allergies, children and teenagers with accelerated growth, being on a weight-loss program, illness, post-surgery, infections and laxatives that hasten food transit.

Recommended daily intake (RDI) figures, promoted by health authorities are doses to prevent diseases like scurvy. Vitamins and minerals work together, so intake needs to be optimal across all nutrients. In light of this, nutritional experts have introduced the concept of the Optimal Daily Allowance (ODA) to ensure the body can deal with the disorders and stresses of modern day living that may require much higher doses.[150] Unfortunately, ODA calculations are much more complex than for measuring RDI, but research is continuing.[151]

If you decide to take a supplement, if possible buy products containing nutrients derived from quality food, or at least in a form that is well absorbed. The high volume of minerals such as magnesium and calcium could mean that more than one tablet is required. Technology in production is evolving, including aerosol and gel formulations to improve stability and absorption and testing to assess need, discussed later.[152] Always read the labels and follow directions on how and when to take products.

CHAPTER 14

You and Your Health

We are often exposed to general, 'blanket statement' guidelines as if one size fits all, but it is not as simple as this as each of us is unique. That is why most health promotions finish with a recommendation to seek specific advice from your health professionals, as they understand your unique individuality.

Even for identical twins living together, varied diets and life experiences make them unique. The key is to appreciate all the available options and apply what works for you, with professional guidance along the way. Just as the squeaky wheel gets the oil, sometimes you need to be an advocate for yourself. Like a woman on the Doctor Oz show who persisted after doctors said her nausea and stomach pain were due to stress, when another doctor found it was stomach cancer.

Your personality

Factors considered in the perception section contribute to each of us having a unique personality that affects our thoughts, determine our attitudes and influence the words we use and the actions we take that become our habits, character and destiny.

Florence Littauer in her book *Personality Plus* suggests we fall into one or two of her four classifications, i.e. powerful choleric, peaceful phlegmatic, popular sanguine and the perfect melancholy.[153] Understanding personality and its effect on our perception of the world (worldview) is critical for good human relationships, so I hope it gets adequate attention in our schools.

Brad Sugars talks about a victor mentality, i.e. someone who is proactive, takes ownership of problems, is accountable and responsible, versus a victim mentality, where people blame others when things go wrong, make excuses and generally are in denial of important issues in their lives. [www.bradsugars.com]

The following acronyms help to remember this, e.g. someone lying in 'bed' **b**laming others, using **e**xcuses and in **d**enial, or someone moving forward, rowing a boat with an 'oar,' displaying **o**wnership, **a**ccountability and **r**esponsibility.

Focus on the glass being half-full, not half-empty. Be a person who sees the ocean, not as a barrier but as an invitation to travel overseas.

Some people won't try new things or take risks out of fear. In *Rich Dad, Poor Dad*, Robert Kiyosaki highlights that some of our best learning in life comes from mistakes we make. He suggests that fear of failing exams at school is entrenched in the minds of some students, holding them back from stepping outside their comfort zone to become entrepreneurs and high achievers.

In fact, after dealing with the basics of life like food and shelter, your life is made up of what you choose to do. Choose to be positive and take on board what Henry Ford said, "If you think you can or if you think you cannot, either way you will be right." Believe in yourself, invest in personal development books and programs, and just do it!

How support can help

Have you ever noticed that most champion sports players have a coach or personal trainer to help them achieve goals? When you think about it, most of us would say it is easier to take a walk regularly with someone else, especially to keep us honest on days when we are tempted to skip it. It makes sense for all of us to have someone to encourage and keep us on track towards our goals, whether a professional coach or simply a like-minded friend.

Ideally it should be someone comfortable saying things that need to be said rather than only what you want to hear, e.g. someone not too '**nice**,' an acronym, developed by business coach Brad Sugars - **n**othing **i**nside of me **c**ares **e**nough (about you) to be frank and honest with you, e.g. "Do you know you have body odour?"[154]

Your coach can help in many ways, including listening to what you say (or do not say), asking questions about where you are and what you want to achieve, finding out what is working for you, what you are willing to sacrifice, and what steps you need to take. They need to pay attention to your needs, be intuitive, non-judgmental, hold you accountable, measure your progress and support you.[155]

Start thinking now about who you want to help you with your health Action Plan, but beware of things like jealous smokers sabotaging those who've given it up, as found in recent research.

In *Did You Spot the Gorilla?* Richard Wiseman describes an experiment where he asks his audience to watch a short film to see how many times a ball is passed. In the film an actor, dressed in a gorilla suit, comes into the scene, thumps his chest and looks at the camera. Typically, half the audience does not see the gorilla, highlighting how easy it is to miss important things when focused on something else like driving a car whilst talking on a hand-held phone.[156] Be sure you are not distracted from important issues in your life; let your coach keep you on track.

The concept of sufferers of similar medical conditions coming together to share knowledge and experiences is both positive and helpful. If you have a disease, ask if a patient-support group exists in your location and think seriously about getting involved.

If none exists, consider starting one up yourself, especially if you find yourself suffering a rare disease that even health practitioners know little about. I am sure you will find health professionals prepared to assist you. Just ask. Some groups operate via a website, allowing sufferers from all parts of the world to share ideas and experiences.

Privacy

Beware of individuals and organisations breaking the laws about your privacy. Do not be afraid to ask to speak to someone privately, should you find yourself in a waiting room or hospital bed and expected to release sensitive information where strangers are able to hear it. In places like pharmacies, ask to discuss personal information in a private area or office, but respect any professional's hesitancy about situations involving the opposite sex. Talk to the New Zealand Privacy Commission if you have any concerns or constructive feedback to offer.[157]

Sometimes privacy laws counter what most would think is fair and reasonable, e.g. a pharmacist found himself in trouble when he innocently issued a family prescription receipt that revealed the daughter was on an oral contraceptive she did not want her parents to know about. In another example, a doctor did not tell parents that their son was suicidal (possibly caused by a medicine he was taking) believing privacy laws prevented it. The teenager subsequently committed suicide.

Be ready for an emergency

To maintain your health, be well prepared for an emergency, that could strike at the most inconvenient time. Check the Civil Defence website [www.getthru.govt.nz] or in some phone books for ideas on disasters like earthquakes and tsunamis.

Keep details of important phone numbers, such as the National Poisons Centre (0800-POISON -764766) and Healthline (0800-611116) on hand. Prepare a getaway kit for evacuation and have a stockpile of survival items and regular medicines to cover a few days.

Act now for yourself and the sake of your family. Remember if a disaster strikes and you are not prepared, you may not be able to access critical items in your house, and emergency services may not be able to get to you for some time. Think about important issues such as adequate petrol in your vehicle, your pets, how to turn off essential services like gas, water and electricity and keeping tools and special equipment like a jack available to lift heavy objects trapping people, etc.

Set up a neighbourhood support network. Find out how on www.ns.org.nz. They are a great way for groups of neighbours to help each other, with members receiving prompt information about emergencies via email. Alternatively, register with Civil Defence for their service.

A doctor on a UK documentary series, *24 Hours in Accident and Emergency* suggests we all could benefit from spending a day observing an emergency department to appreciate how fragile we are and to encourage us to pay more attention to those we love, rather than the hectic lifestyle most lead today. This might stimulate more of the public to do a first aid course. He also suggested that people doing CPR (cardio-pulmonary resuscitation) concentrate on doing 100 chest compressions per minute, hard enough to compress the chest about a third of its thickness, i.e. 'hard and fast.'

For children and babies, do two breaths for every 30 compressions but do not worry about the breathing for adults, unless someone else is available to help. A paramedic friend stresses the key points of CPR are to get the patient onto a hard flat surface, if possible. Don't worry about trying to find a pulse, position yourself close to their body and keep your arms straight.

If an portable AED (automated external defibrillator) is available, connect it to the patient and follow the machine's verbal commands, as it is virtually in charge, i.e. it checks to see if it needs to shock the patient and tells operators when to continue CPR etc. The machines are easy to use and go hand in hand with CPR to greatly increase the chances of survival.

When ringing the emergency number '111' in New Zealand and connected to the ambulance service, you're usually speaking to a trained officer who can give you advice and mental support until an ambulance arrives. Note too that the phone remains connected until the crisis is over, to avoid unintentional disconnection.

Technology now allows patients to wear panic buttons that connect to emergency services and even send texts or emails to support contacts. Some are able to indicate where the sender is through global positioning systems (GPS). If you have a panic button, check to see if it is waterproof and wear it at all times including in the shower. Murphy's Law tells us problems will usually arise when we least expect it, and are not prepared.

Technology is great, but sometimes there are downsides of a change e.g. some portable home telephones rely on power, so are useless in a power failure.

A pandemic is an epidemic of infectious disease that is widespread, usually across continents. Should one occur, keep up with media reports on what to do. General advice is to wash your hands often and thoroughly and stay home. Keep a supply of gloves and quality facemasks to hand, and remember even those showing no symptoms at the time of contact could still be spreading infections.

Insurance

Some time ago I had a blood test, which suggested a colonoscopy and gastroscopy would be helpful to eliminate serious disease. My doctor referred me to a surgeon, whose first question was whether I had private hospital insurance as he said the wait in the public system was nine months, whereas he could do the job privately in five weeks.

Knowing the potential seriousness of the situation, I decided to go private. Not long after, I discovered another patient of the surgeon had the same procedures in a public hospital within eight weeks, at no cost to him. My procedure cost me $1,700 because my insurance policy only covered $500 of the $2,200 expense. I sent the surgeon a letter asking for an explanation. He phoned back to say that waiting times change all the time.

The moral of the story is to read your insurance policy carefully, checking for exclusions and find ways to see if the information you're getting is correct.

An insurance broker confirmed that prices of medical procedures are probably higher than they should be because, with insurance, patients do not question charges as much as they would if they were paying the bill. Insurance premiums are climbing steadily, with more people questioning their need for cover. A good exercise is to estimate what your insurance will cost you over the next ten years and weigh up the chances you will need that amount of money for private health work, not covered by the public system. Surgery charges vary, so it pays to shop around.

Organ and blood donation

Around the world many patients are on waiting lists for donor organs. To reduce low rates of donation, some countries require people to opt out if they do not want to be donors. Think seriously about the power you possess to help someone in their hour of need, including life-saving blood.

Men and health

Typically men are not as good as women when it comes to being pro-active with their health. I have to confess, for instance, that when I was unwell and busy with our pharmacy, it took me some time to go and see Dr Higgins, the wholistic GP who solved a problem that my regular doctor could not. If it had not been for my wife it is likely I would have taken even longer to seek help and find out all the good he could do for me.

Most men tend to think they are 'bulletproof' and that health issues will not affect them, as reflected in a USA colon cancer screening program which showed men were under-represented in presentation, but over-represented in both polyp and cancer detection.[158]

One initiative to draw attention to men's health issues - and we need more - is 'MOvember,' where men grow a moustache for the month of November each year.[159]

Prostate problems

Symptoms of prostate problems include a weak urine stream, getting up to more than once at night to urinate, frequent urination during the day (even though little urine is present), an urgent need to urinate and difficulty getting urine to flow. These symptoms may indicate treatable conditions such as benign prostatic hyperplasia (BPH), but may also be a clue to prostate cancer, which kills about 550 men in New Zealand each year. In our pharmacy we regularly issued a urine score sheet for men to complete and show their doctor.

Whilst not conclusive, doctors use a digital rectal examination (DRE), combined with a PSA blood test to check for prostate cancer. With low-grade prostate cancer, research suggests it may be prudent to focus on active surveillance rather than rush in with treatment that may have adverse effects, including impotence and incontinence.[160]

Sun exposure

Over-exposure to the sun with UVA (ultraviolet light, wavelength group A) causes skin ageing and skin cancer and UVB (group B) causes burning and skin cancer. Whilst the sun has its benefits (as discussed), it is important to control exposure, especially with rising skin cancer rates in New Zealand.

Experts say it is prudent to go to the beach in the morning or late afternoon and to seek shade whenever possible, but remember that air scatters UV light, so you can still burn under shade. How much exposure we need is not clear, or well-studied. Definitive guidelines are difficult, due to variation in skin colour, atmospheric ozone 'holes,' seasonal UV ratings and location on earth, which affects the angle of the sun and the intensity of exposure. Note too that not all sunglasses protect eyes from ultraviolet light.

The main intention is to avoid sunburn as this increases the risk of skin cancer. Consider broad-brimmed hats, instead of caps that give little ear and neck protection. The **sun protection factor** (SPF) gives an indication of protection from UVB, but not UVA. An SPF of 30 provides individual protection for 30 times what it normally takes for reddening of the skin (burn time), assuming it is used according to the manufacturer's instructions and not sweated or washed off. Reapplication does not extend exposure time.

Aim for products with an SPF of 30 or more, but remember going from an SPF 30 to 50 means minimal extra protection. To my knowledge, there are currently no international standards for UVA protection. Buy broad-spectrum protection (UVA and UVB) products and follow storage conditions and expiry dates to ensure efficacy.

An adult needs about 10ml (2 teaspoonfuls) for the face and arms and 35ml for full body coverage. A study of beach volleyball players, found the majority used less than a quarter of the recommended amount.[161] As it is not easy to see areas missed, apply two coats as you would to paint a house, ideally with a spray or a lotion that spreads easily. Apply sunscreen 15 minutes before going into the sun and reapply according to the manufacturer's instructions.

Zinc and titanium oxide provide a physical broad-spectrum block, but beware of products made with tiny nano-particles that may be absorbed, the significance of which is not yet apparent, as more research is needed.

Researchers have noted a rise in the incidence of melanoma even with the increasing use of sunscreens, suggesting that they may not give as good protection as first thought. However some patients get melanomas in places not normally exposed to sunlight and absorbed sunscreens may increase free radicals. Take extra care if you have already had skin cancer. New Zealand dermatologist, Dr Marius Rademaker, stresses the hazards of tanning lamps, with a recent UK study finding they increase the risk of skin cancer by up to 75%.[162] [www.cancernz.org.nz]

Alcohol

Alcohol contains seven calories (30 kJ) per gram and has a range of mental effects including relaxation, loss of co-ordination, addiction and stimulation or sadness (depending on one's environment). It can also weaken the immune system, cause dehydration, and liver damage.

Billions are spent each year around the world treating alcohol-related problems including heart disease, brain damage, cancers (especially breast bowel and prostate), liver disease, domestic violence, crime, financial and productivity losses, weight gain, industrial mishaps and traffic crashes (many of which are not 'accidents' per se). Ironically, some RTD (ready to drink) products can be cheaper than bottled water.

Whether alcohol has any health benefits, as some would like to think, is controversial. In fact it is listed as a cancer causing agent by WHO. Any benefits from poly-phenol antioxidants in red wine are minimal, as the concentration is low so it is more realistic to get these from superfoods. Whilst recommendations vary, and there is no 'safe' level, authorities suggest no more than one standard drink a day, less than you might be pouring now, as you should get around six standard glasses of wine from a bottle.

Alcohol can cause people to be overconfident and more likely to crash when they drink and drive, especially if they have not been eating at the same time. Because the effects of alcohol on the individual are highly variable, breath and blood testing levels are not particularly reliable as an indicator of impairment. Surveys indicate many people are uncertain of the amount of alcohol it takes to affect their ability to drive, suggesting a need for other sobriety tests such as walking a straight line.

Some of us have a gene that enhances the effect of alcohol and increases our chances of addiction, so a logical suggestion is for authorities to test first-time drunk drivers for this gene.

Most authorities say to avoid alcohol during pregnancy because of the risk of the child developing foetal alcohol syndrome, which can cause brain damage. The New Zealand Doctor website reports that 'after many years of lobbying, the Australian and New Zealand Council on Food Regulation will now look at introducing appropriate labelling about the risks of drinking alcohol during pregnancy in 2014.' One has to wonder why such logical actions take so long.

Caffeine

Caffeine is a stimulant that works by muscling in on spaces in your brain normally reserved for the natural sedative adenosine. The effects of caffeine vary from person to person. The upside is that a small amount of caffeine improves mental and physical performance, reaction time, and even mood, but larger doses can cause anxiety, restlessness, irritability, sleeplessness, headaches, stomach upsets, and nausea with exceptionally high intakes linked with osteoporosis, high blood pressure, adverse cholesterol levels, heart problems, even death.

Addiction to energy drinks containing caffeine (guarana) and high amounts of sugar is a big problem, especially in young adults. Maximum dose is about 400mg per day.

Sleep

Research suggests the typical human being needs around 7 to 9 hours of continuous sleep every 24 hours. Inadequate sleep is associated with increased susceptibility to infections, slowed growth, enlarged prostate, diabetes, high blood pressure, stroke, weight gain (through reduced metabolism), and increased cortisol and appetite. Some researchers liken the effects of inadequate sleep to a hangover, resulting in reduced learning and increased road crashes. Contrary to popular belief, snoring is not always a sign of 'deep' sleep, especially if the person actually stops breathing for a short time, which could indicate sleep apnoea that needs investigation.

Insomnia is the medical term to describe an inability to get adequate, quality deep sleep, which may result in resorting to sleeping pills. Typically this happens in hospitals. Beware of this becoming a habit back in the community, as some can cause personality changes and addiction. Consider options like passionflower and valerian.

Lack of sleep may be due to stress, lack of melatonin, or low magnesium levels, which can be checked with a blood test. Other causes include heartburn, through eating too much close to bedtime, especially chocolate or citrus; chronic pain; some medicines, and too high a bedroom temperature.

Ironically, some people have disturbed sleep because of low blood sugars during the night, so a healthy snack before bedtime can work for them. Foods that may assist sleep because they contain tryptophan include milk, banana, almonds, tuna on wholegrain toast and yoghurt.[163] Achieve better sleep through a routine, pre-bed ritual to get your thoughts and atmosphere right. Avoid daytime naps and limit stimulants like caffeine after 5pm.

Whilst on the subject of sleep, let me give you a few tips about getting out of bed, taught to me by the Morgan Clinic in Tauranga. Roll onto your side, facing the side of the bed. Push your upper body upright, using your upper arm across the body. Drop your legs to the floor and stand. This procedure may lessen your chances of back problems, caused by suddenly jumping out of bed and the risk of twisting the spine in the process.

Depression and suicide

John Kirwan with his book *All Blacks Don't Cry* and his regular TV ads has done much to raise awareness of depression that may lead to suicide. Over 500 people commit suicide in New Zealand each year, many more than die in the quad bike incidents that get much more attention. In 2013 a coroner raised concerns about 'ongoing failures of mental health support systems to prevent suicides.'

The more open we are about suicide, the more likely people are to realise that someone they know may need help. The critical thing is to be pro-active, even to the point of asking direct questions such as "Are you considering taking your life?" Actively help them get treatment or tell someone who can deal with your suspicions. Comments like 'pull your socks up' are definitely unhelpful. In New Zealand a free phone support system called Lifeline is available (0800 LIFELINE or 0800-543354.)[164]

Do not prejudge: you might not know all the facts. For example, recent research links a 50% increase in suicide rates in those infected with *Toxoplasma gondii*, a common parasite in cats that affects about a third of the world population without external symptoms. It is capable of causing other serious health conditions, especially in those who are pregnant, or whose immune system is weak. A blood test to detect the parasite is available.

Toxins

Toxicity can be acute, build up over time and is often overlooked and difficult to define. In 2011 a mysterious illness in Germany was tracked to sprays used on cotton crops and poisons in the dyes used during manufacture, highlighting how challenging it can be to trace and prove toxicity. It may be in the air we breathe and in our water supplies. Bearing this in mind, we need to be cautious about 'fracking,' a term used in the oil industry to describe the use of high-pressure water and chemicals to fracture soil when drilling, which could contaminate surface water. Some countries have banned it.

Infections account for millions of deaths around the world each year, e.g. malaria, spread by mosquitoes, is endemic in 106 nations and kills one child every thirty seconds in Africa. The chemical DDT is effective in controlling the breeding grounds and is still in use today. This is an example where a toxin is the lesser of two evils, so long as it is well controlled, which was not the case years ago when the risk of environmental contamination through indiscriminate use attracted widespread attention after biologist Rachel Carson published *Silent Spring*.

A vaccine for malaria looks to be on the horizon, as does a new quick, cheaper and easier method of diagnosis being developed in Japan by M. Kataoka.

The website www.breastcancerfund.org provides details of links between heart disease, diabetes and cancer to chemicals like bisphenol-A (BPA), a hormone disruptor used to make plastic liners in some cans and other food containers.[165] New Zealand health authorities say levels in our food are 'low and safe,' yet the *Healthy Food Guide* advises 'do not refill bottled water containers for more than four weeks, and consider glass or BPA-free plastic for baby feeding bottles.'

A report in 2010 from the FDA raised concerns regarding exposure of foetuses, infants and young children to BPA. In September 2010, Canada became the first country to declare it a toxic substance and both the European Union and Canada have banned it in baby bottles.

Concerns are emerging about the toxic effects of a chemical called Corexit, used to disperse oil from ocean spills; some countries ban it. Even dishwashing detergent can cause health problems if not rinsed off before drying. [www.biocerasa.co.za] Toxins may also be present in cosmetics.[166] [167]

We need to be ever vigilant as evidenced by the dust from the destruction of the twin towers in New York after 9/11. Initially declared safe by authorities it was subsequently found to contain heavy metals, with links to an ongoing serious lung condition.

Many illnesses are associated with toxins and allergies, so if you have unresolved medical conditions, consult a specialist.

There are many means by which we can reduce environmental pollution. Some are as simple as asking smokers to carry a metal container to collect their butts, rather than dropping them on the ground or flicking them out of car windows where they end up polluting harbours and streams. In other examples, the New Zealand dairy co-operative Fonterra plans to stop collecting milk from farms without waterways fenced off, to reduce water pollution, and dairy farmers are establishing effluent storage facilities to reduce runoff, when soils are too wet.

The value of regular check-ups

Take a moment to think about how many cars you've owned to date. At my seminars, the average among the audience is ten. Now imagine if you could only have one car in your lifetime. Would that make a difference to how you looked after it?

You only have one body that works hard to keep you alive and well. It contains around 100 trillion cells, most of which are replaced annually and your blood travels 19,000 kilometres per day. Your red blood cells make a quarter of a million trips around your body before they're replaced.

Your heart pumps about 70ml of blood about 70 times a minute, i.e. about 7,000 litres per day. By age 80 your heart will have pumped over 200 million litres of blood around your body with a pressure akin to a tight squeeze on a tennis ball. After what it does for you, it deserves special attention.

I find it hard to fathom why people know how important it is to put the right fuel in the tank of their car and regularly check the oil, etc., yet think nothing about putting rubbish food (fuel) in their stomach (tank) and expect to stay healthy.

There is no shortage of research showing the benefits of a healthy lifestyle to prevent many diseases, e.g. the *British Journal of Cancer* reported in 2011 that 40% of cancers are associated with lifestyle choices. This is a reminder to favour prevention before cure, with the treatment of symptoms as a last resort. Think of it as being a property investor in for the long haul, with no expectation of a return on investment for years.

Just like the consequences of a car running out of oil, the earlier a problem is detected and dealt with the better, e.g. the Breast Cancer Foundation of New Zealand says 95% of breast cancer patients are alive after five years if detected from mammograms, compared to 73% when cancer is detected as a lump (lymph nodes also should be checked.)[168] Alternative detection methods are also available, or coming.

A good maintenance (check-up) program for your body is important as many diseases do not show symptoms in the early stages, e.g. autopsies of young soldiers, killed in the Korean War showed 75% had a degree of blood vessel narrowing and plaque build-up.

New Zealand has one of the highest rates of malignant melanoma in the world hence the need for regular check-ups, ideally with adequate technology such as the SIAscope, developed in the United Kingdom for improved detection. In years to come, our existing detection systems will be regarded as crude, but we need to make the most of what we have today.

Just as a car needs regular servicing to prevent damage and breakdowns, so too does your body, especially keeping the big picture in mind. Listen to your body for subtle changes that may signal challenges, and do not lapse into a false sense of security, as check-ups are not a substitute for a healthy lifestyle.

Family history

In 2013, Angelina Jolie underwent a double mastectomy operation after the discovery that she carried the BRCA1 or BRAC2 gene, associated with an increased risk of developing breast or ovarian cancer, especially if other relatives are affected. Her story attracted worldwide media coverage, alerting many women to something they probably did not know about. Now we are discovering the genes might be associated with some male diseases.

Whilst watching the Dr Oz show it occurred to me that this heart surgeon is doing a great job helping his audience of millions to stay healthy, including the importance of knowing about serious diseases or conditions in your own family history. This is especially important for conditions that are hard to detect like pancreatic cancer, where back pain could give a clue.

Another is ovarian cancer, where symptoms that include bloating, bowel problems, constipation and haemorrhoids mean women should promptly consult their doctor.

The Centers for Disease Control and Prevention (CDC) in the USA has a plan to prevent one million heart attacks in a 5-year period. One strategy is to get everyone to take a serious look at their family history, something they say few people do.

Start right now, beginning with your parents, siblings and ancestors. Look in records and make enquiries at family reunions. Realise some conditions had different titles in the past, e.g. 'wheezy bronchitis' for asthma and 'mental breakdown' for depression. Collect details including at what age they occurred, as this may give a clue to risk.

Report your findings to your doctor as soon as possible as this could increase your chances of living a longer, healthier life and be a gift to those you love and who love you. That said, research suggests the environment plays an important role in whether certain genes are activated or not.

General issues

There are many things you can do to keep an eye on your health, e.g. to protect your eyes as much as possible have regular tests to assess your vision and the presence of diseases like glaucoma; note and report changes in moles; or stiffness, pain, or coffee-coloured bowel motions that could indicate a stomach bleed.

Some health tests are readily available privately, e.g. a taste test to give an indication of zinc levels in the body is available at some pharmacies and health food shops. The *Readers Digest* published the following list of checks you can do at home, with the proviso that you discuss the results with your health practitioner:[169]

- A wheeze or cough. A point to note here is that shortness of breath may be due to heart failure leading to a build-up of fluid in the lungs interfering with breathing.
- A pale palm crease may indicate low iron, especially in women.
- Check your pulse and note any irregularities that might indicate heart problems.
- Review the diabetes risk factors: older, male, sibling with the disease, high blood sugar, urinary frequency, low fruit and vegetable consumption and less than three hours of exercise per week.
- Check how well you can bend and stretch.
- Act if stomach measurement is over 94cm for men and over 80cm for women.

- Take a depression questionnaire test. Also be aware European scientists at MedUni in Vienna are working on a blood test to detect the condition.

One day in our pharmacy my wife Judy noted a mole on the back of a customer's neck that proved to be a malignant melanoma. Fortunately, early detection gave a good outcome for a grateful woman. This is a reminder how important it is to be on the lookout all the time and to be aware of tools like the '**ABCDE**' of a melanoma that can be a good trigger for action i.e. is the 'mole' **a**symmetric, are the **b**orders irregular, is it **c**oloured, is the **d**iameter greater than a pencil and is it **e**levated (raised).

Ears and hearing

Over half a million New Zealanders suffer some degree of hearing impairment. To protect your hearing, avoid noisy environments, wear earmuffs and especially beware of playing music too loudly through headphones and noisy toys, especially when held up to the ears. 85-decibel noise levels can damage ears, and a power drill may be this loud, with circular saws and lawnmowers louder. Be aware of deafness that might be impeding early childhood development.

Medical tests and screening

Once a new test is developed, experts decide on the expected range of values in a typical population. They then test a random group and graph the results as a normal frequency distribution, known as a 'bell curve' (shown at right) where most people have a value around the centre.

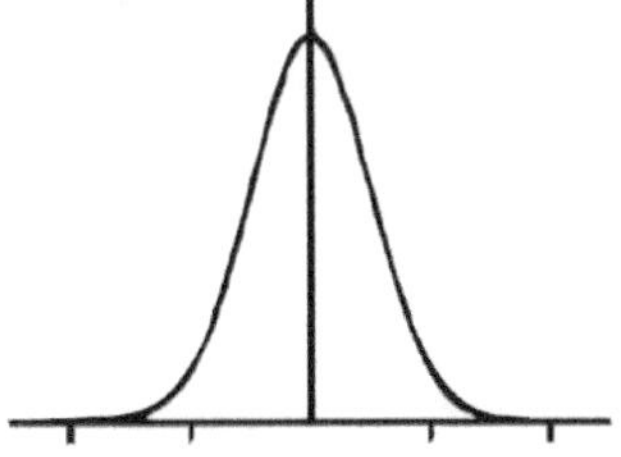

Ongoing monitoring continues to ensure they reflect reality and can be adjusted accordingly. In fact, some doctors now suggest the New Zealand upper limit for thyroid stimulating hormone (TSH) is too high, meaning some patients could be suffering unnecessarily with lethargy, weight gain, hair loss, etc., through an underactive thyroid. As well, a number of conditions may affect results, highlighting the importance of looking at the big picture i.e. tests and patient presentation.

My last selenium blood test result was 1.55 micromoles/L. My doctor's nurse rang me in a bit of a panic to say I was toxic. Whilst the reference range in New Zealand is 0.45-1.4 micromoles/L (and the average blood level is 1.1 micromoles/L), a review published in *The Lancet* medical journal, by

Prof M. Rayman (March 2012) recommends a range of 1.6-1.9 micromoles/L, so according to her, my level was actually low!

A range of medical tests is available, including many to assess a newborn's susceptibility to diseases. Results trigger action, or let parents and caregivers know what they are susceptible to and what precautions they can take to reduce their risk.

Some tests are subsidised by governments and insurance companies. In fact, some insurance companies are happy to pay for check-ups and reward clients for healthy activities.

In some cases, laboratories stop doing a test if a government subsidy is withdrawn, meaning you might need to shop around. Tests for many aspects of health continue to be developed, including the emergence of specialist laboratories providing tests to ascertain vitamin and mineral needs. Some even provide supplements, based on individual DNA test results. The cost and availability will likely improve over time as more take up the opportunity. For more information start with www.biolab.co.uk. Alternative tests include applied kinesiology.

Decisions about health are often about degrees, rather than certainty, e.g. not a case of either 'my mammogram will be normal and I don't have to worry about breast cancer, or it will not be and I will die.' As well as this, it is virtually impossible to measure anything with 100% accuracy, e.g. the 'Hawkeye' system (in tennis) has an error of plus or minus 3.5mm and when measuring a liquid the error is plus or minus half a graduation mark. Ideally, all measurements should indicate the degree of accuracy. With medical tests, there will be some false positives and false negatives.

Even though there are 3,000 new cases of prostate cancer per year in New Zealand (a quarter fatal), there is no screening program as experts say the test is not sensitive enough to differentiate between low-grade cancers and aggressive high-risk cases that could expose those with insignificant cancers to unnecessary anxiety.

Doctors select medical tests they want done from lists on computers, or printed forms. Whilst the incidence is low, errors may occur. These may be where a test is accidently omitted, wrong containers are used, equipment fails or a laboratory mixes up samples, as in the case of a woman who received results about her 'prostate.' A local laboratory is currently installing a 'state of the art' computer tracking system to reduce errors.

Errors can occur if patients do not comply with conditions, e.g. there was a time when blood for a cholesterol test was required to be taken in the morning, before any food, however research now shows this is unnecessary. Because single tests can be wrong, trends are generally more reliable.

Measurements as basic as blood pressure (BP) can be wrong through faulty equipment or operator technique, e.g. a larger cuff is needed for a large arm, or the phenomenon called 'white coat syndrome' where blood pressure can be high in a doctor's surgery (due to anxiety, etc.), yet normal at other times. A UK study in 2012 found patients treated inappropriately for high blood pressure because of this, prompting moves for portable monitoring to determine actual readings.

Some tests are part of public screening programs that involve consideration of many issues, including cost/benefit ratio, what age groups to include, test accuracy, and likely uptake by the public. Even targeting direct relatives of patients with particular diseases may be useful. There will always be ideas about other diseases that warrant action, e.g. hemochromatosis (excess iron) that injures body organs and can be fatal unless detected in time. It often comes down to priority and available funding.[170]

Some years ago in our pharmacy, we stocked an **OTC** 'over the counter' product to detect blood in faeces (stools) that might indicate bowel cancer. This is curable if discovered early, yet kills about four times as many people as die on New Zealand roads. Whilst we promoted the product enthusiastically and sold it for just $10, we could not get many customers motivated enough to buy it.

Whilst I am sure people did grasp the merits of the test, they were not keen on what was required, i.e. dropping a piece of paper into the toilet bowl after a bowel motion and looking for a colour change. A pilot screening program for 50 to 75 year olds with a new product is underway (2013) in parts of Auckland. I hope people take this seriously and see that pharmacists are in an ideal position to be involved in screening programs like this.

Sometimes health departments focus on areas that need special attention with publicity campaigns, etc. One example is rheumatic heart disease that affects some people through a streptococcal throat infection and which is killing around 145 - mainly children - each year in New Zealand. BLIS K12 throat guard boost may be helpful to reduce the incidence.

What tests are right for you?

In an ideal world, you might expect to have absolutely everything checked, like aeronautical engineers preparing a jetliner for a test flight. However, when it comes to your body it gets complicated because of many factors including cost, knowledge, availability, reliability and the worldview of patients; and professionals, trying to get the balance right between a need for tests and clinical judgment.

Professionals may not do certain tests because they are confident about a diagnosis (yet could be wrong); pressure from government to keep costs down, or are off their 'radar screen' through ignorance (10% of lung cancer occurs in non-smokers), or because they are not subsidised. It is a good idea to tell your doctor if you are happy to pay for unsubsidised tests, but be aware prices may vary e.g. selenium and vitamin D.

In the end there will always be discussion about what tests to do. Ask good probing questions to satisfy yourself that your check up is exhaustive and in line with the latest standards. Do not dismiss things you put down to 'old age,' without discussion.

Some medical imaging has led to more risks than first thought, e.g. research (2012) from the UK suggests children who have multiple CT scans by age 15 have a high risk of developing a brain tumour or leukaemia in later life. Ask questions. "Why do I need this? Will it change therapy? Am I getting the lowest dose possible and can we document the dosage on my records?[171]

When a drop of blood is required for tests like a blood glucose, the side of the finger should be used, where thinner and less sensitive skin makes the job easier and less painful.

Some other key points to consider in a consultation with your doctor are as follows:

- General blood test that may include insulin resistance and haemoglobin A1C to detect fluctuations in blood sugar levels over the previous three months.
- Intolerance tests such as gluten and lactose.
- Hormone tests including testosterone, progesterone and DHEA.
- Inflammation tests, i.e. ratio of omega-6 to omega-3 i.e. AA (arachidonic acid)/EPA, and C reactive protein.
- Tests for vitamin, mineral and antioxidant levels, especially those discussed in the deficiency section.
- Risk factors for disease, including your family history.
- Consider removing make-up, as discussed.
- Could referral to a complementary practitioner be helpful?
- Ensure you are on appropriate screening programs, e.g. cervical, breast cancer and for men, a prostate test (PSA) and digital rectal examination (DRE).
- Be aware of new ideas from around the world, e.g. Dr Arthur Agatston has invented a 'coronary calcium scan' that he says helps detect those at risk of a heart attack or stroke.
- With HIV incidence rising in the heterosexual world and a lack of public health reminders plus a degree of complacency about the risks, a test for this might be appropriate.

- Other relevant tests, e.g. a carotid ultrasound eye scan to detect amyloid protein associated with Alzheimer's disease; skin examination for cancerous moles; hearing, sight, glaucoma and memory tests.
- Blood-level tests are available to monitor side effects and effectiveness of some medicines.

When and how often

In general, heart disease tends to affect men earlier than women, so start testing men around 45 years of age and women around 55. Certain ethnics groups and those with a family history or other personal risk factors should have screening earlier.

How often a reassessment is done will depend on your health professional, with increased frequency with higher risks. Dental checks are recommended every six months.

Many a time I have heard someone say, "I had a blood test and doctor says everything is okay," which may not be the case, due to errors as discussed. Some doctors send patients results, or list them on websites, which is great to get involvement and track trends. Dr Higgins always sent me a copy with detailed comments, yet today, this is still not routine. If you have not heard, do not assume all is okay and ring to check. Ideally your doctor will have a reminder on their computer for ongoing tests, especially important if your regular doctor is away.

All the above is rational, according to our current thinking. However, in the year 2000 heart specialists noted that a significant number of the population have an unexpected heart attack or stroke, suggesting our systems are not as sophisticated as some think.

Out of this observation has arisen an idea to mass medicate the majority of the population over 55 years of age with low dose aspirin and medicines to control cholesterol and blood pressure. Research suggests this action could reduce the incidence of heart attacks and strokes by over 50%, and higher if combined with a healthy lifestyle. Trials are currently underway in India. Dr S. Holt tells the full story in his book *Miracle Pill*.[172]

CHAPTER 15

Health Care in the Future

In 2011 health professionals published a letter in the *New Zealand Medical Journal*, expressing concern at the rapid rise in the incidence of diabetes and the need to do more to deal with this serious problem. This and other health crises suggest there is no better time than now to take a long hard look at how we do things in the health services at the political, bureaucratic and personal level. From there we need to develop a co-ordinated plan, based on what works, what does not and how to learn from mistakes and move forward, without reinventing the wheel.

Wholistic 'big picture' health

It's human nature to seek a 'quick fix' for health problems, like taking a pill for cholesterol, yet continuing on with poor lifestyle habits. There are plenty of so-called 'magic bullets' on the market, but beware of unproven or risky products marketed with an eye to profit, not your health. Just as many diseases develop over time, preventative long-term treatment usually take some time to work, so quick fixes may be helpful in the interim, e.g. blood pressure control with medicines as a stepping-stone to an altered lifestyle.

"Keeping the 'big picture' in mind means we don't get bogged down in the fine detail," says cardiologist Professor T. Campbell at St Vincent's Hospital in Sydney. He suggests "a lot of medical studies are focusing on small aspects of health that reveal little about the big picture, and cause us to not progress as quickly as we should."[173] I am sure the same applies to personal health.

I dream of a future with more and more health practitioners from diverse backgrounds working together in patients' best interests. The movement is gaining traction with the Cancer Society of New Zealand now suggesting a more collaborative approach needs to apply to the treatment of cancer. More doctors now have complementary skills like acupuncture or incorporate complementary professionals into their practice.

Over the years, I have seen many people jump to false conclusions or make bad decisions 'cherry-picking' information out of context. This often happened because they did not have sufficient background knowledge to appreciate the big picture. In some cases they put others in this position e.g. asking a librarian friend if their prescribed medicines were good for them; and poor language skills due to an ignorance of grammar.

Expense prioritisation

In *Heathcheque* economists Gareth Morgan and Geoff Simmons surveyed different health systems through a series of interviews with health administrators, professionals, patients and the public.[174] They found the big drivers for expenditure included salaries and wages, high cost technology and the emerging impact of baby boomers.

The authors also found some unrealistic expectations of what the health system can deliver and that a significant part of health budgets are spent on care for people in the last phase of life, with family, friends and health professionals pushing for action ahead of most patients.

We pay taxes in exchange for products and services rendered by government. Given the money actually belongs to the people, it is important we keep an eye on priorities, to ensure they are appropriate. Whilst productivity in the New Zealand health system has been relatively good, costs are rising at an ever-increasing rate, with affordability being a challenge that has led to more rationing.

In 2012 government health expenditure in New Zealand was about $14 billion, 9% of gross domestic product and predicted to double in the next forty years. Money always has alternate uses, making it difficult to make decisions, especially in the health field. Imagine how much easier it would be if humans had a dollar value like a prize bull.

To complicate things, many medical treatments have benefits that only just outweigh the risks or costs, e.g. if we treat 100 people with a 20% risk of a heart attack we might save 20, but if we treat 500 with a 10% risk we might save 50. Clearly the cost-to-benefit ratio plays a big role in where the line is drawn.

Costing expenses down to individual patients may improve the '**system**' (**s**aves **y**ou **s**tress, **t**ime, **e**nergy and **m**oney). This approach might be a way to deal with government silos where actions in one department results in problems elsewhere. For instance, the government sets Pharmac's budget, yet devolves decision-making and rationing to them, with little accountability of both parties, because they can blame the other party if things go wrong. Those with rare diseases needing expensive medicines that are not subsidised by Pharmac will attest to this.

Some suggest 'healthy foods' should be exempt from goods and services tax, whereas others say it is better to tax 'unhealthy' food at around 20%, which is seen as the level to make a difference. However, as discussed earlier, it is difficult to put food into 'good' and 'bad' categories, as it depends on a number of issues, including the context in which it is used. Having said that, a New Zealand survey in 2013 found respondents favoured a tax on 'unhealthy' food, so this may be what it takes to get people to change their lifestyle habits here. [http://www.3news.co.nz/tvshows/vote/the-vote-is-it-time-to-tax-unhealthy-food-2013032715]

It will be interesting to see the outcomes of overseas experiences taxing certain foods, e.g. in Denmark high saturated fat; in France soft drinks; in Norway sugar and chocolate, and in the UK sugary drinks and plans to limit fast food outlets near schools. Mexico is planning a tax of 8% on junk food. Alternatively authorities in Hampden, Massachusetts, USA are trialling tax credits for purchases of fruit and vegetables.

Accountability

Our family doctor never charged for follow-up visits if his treatment hadn't worked, yet, typically we see health providers focussed on high patient turnover on a 'fee for service' basis without any guarantee of results. Just as customers would not pay a tradesman for faulty workmanship, why is it not the same for health providers? True, medicine is not as black and white as fixing a leaking roof, but the idea is worth considering.

I was surprised when I arrived in New Zealand in 1985 to find that pharmacists did not have professional insurance to cover medical misadventure, as in Western Australia, where my cover was $5 million. I was told not to worry as professionals cannot be sued in New Zealand, where misadventure may be covered by ACC. My immediate thought was this approach was likely to reduce accountability and lower professional standards, and I have seen a number of examples of this.

In 2011 ACC had 1.67 million claims for home injuries costing $300 million. One wonders how much this would drop if people had to pay if they were negligent. Taking this a step further, should ACC cover dangerous sports and activities where participants do not wear protective gear?

An overseas visitor had a hip replacement in New Zealand through ACC. He offered to pay, but they refused, emphasising he was 'entitled.' Obviously, some people find it easy to spend other people's - taxpayers' - money.

Revelations in 2012 of lax privacy procedures and a focus on getting long-term cases off ACC through staff bonus payments has led some advisers to suggest it is time we opened the system to competition and the right to sue for incompetence. The key would be to have lawyers paid on a time basis, not on percentages of large claims, as seen overseas.

A health professional I know justifies his smoking by saying, "I have paid enough taxes to cover the costs of any smoking-related health issues I develop." His stance begs the question of how we can achieve accountability through society from the politicians (and the systems they create) to managers and workers in that system, right down to individuals who cause health problems?

Proving cause and effect is difficult, but as we do not have a bottomless pit of money to throw at health issues, we need to look at what is fair and reasonable. This includes patients who do not turn up for public hospital appointments without good reason, highlighting another opportunity for accountability of those who are blasé about free services and deny access to others. Just like a 'free' (subsidised by the government) first aid course I attended where, instead of collecting a bond, to ensure enrolees turned up, the course was half-full and one wonders if this affected the contractor's payment.

Lateral thinking for answers

I have a challenge for you. Join all nine dots (at right) in four straight lines, without lifting your pen off the paper. (Solution at end of the section.) Now, have you ever thought how an invention seems so simple you wonder why you had not thought of it first, like the 'food truck chef' developing healthier fast food?

Many innovations evolve from lateral 'outside the square,' thinking, a concept developed by Edward De Bono. Using techniques such as brainstorming, different, and dramatic ideas, known as paradigm shifts, often emerge.

As an example, software writers in France developed a computer program to control a fleet of delivery trucks, based on observations of beehive activities. There is no 'boss' telling the bees what to do, but some sort of 'system' based on information gathered by individuals.

The moral of this story is that it took thinking 'outside the square' to recognise that a 'bottom-up' approach, based on what was happening at the individual truck level, was superior to a traditional 'top down' approach. Discarding pre-conceived ideas and thinking laterally, I am sure there are many solutions to current health challenges beyond the ideas that follow.

In *Freakonomics*, authors Dubner and Levitt noted legalised abortion was associated with a drop in crime, probably due to fewer unwanted babies being born in sub-standard environments. Wellington's free ambulance service has upskilled staff to treat more patients at home, rather than carting them off to an already overloaded hospital system. The Polypill idea, previously discussed, has some merit in preventing heart attacks and strokes, however, conventional thinking means it is unlikely to come to New Zealand anytime soon.

Now consider how we might deal with conflicts of interest, like governments collecting taxes from the sale of health hazard products such as cigarettes and alcohol. Then we have the issue of New Zealand politicians, elected for three-year terms, tending to focus on achieving a return on expenditure as soon as possible to satisfy voters and get back into power, conflicting with cost-effective prevention strategies that may take years to show benefits. Longer terms of office (with built-in safeguards) may be the answer.

An ex-politician suggests some government administration staff are busy doing jobs they cling to and justify vehemently, even though they do not contribute much to the 'big picture.' Ironically, that person's government allowed the public service bureaucracy to expand dramatically.

Sometimes the focus is on efficiency (doing things right) at the expense of effectiveness (doing the right thing.) e.g. are 21 District Health Boards (more responsible to the Ministry of Health than the communities they represent) effective when you consider the costs, duplication of tasks, signage, varying standards and rationing etc. involved? For a country as small as New Zealand, with high infrastructural costs per head of population, economies of scale are important to get good value for money.

Whilst some will laugh, the producers of the long-running New Zealand television series Shortland Street say the program deals with current health issues, so health administrators may find good ideas here.

The average stay in hospital in New Zealand is shorter than Australia and Japan. Could this be because we are discharging patients too early, in an effort to create good key performance indicators (KPI) for bureaucrats to look good in the eyes of politicians, at the expense of patients? Such was the case of a man discharged from hospital soon after having his medicines altered, only to be readmitted by ambulance in the early hours of the next morning, much to the chagrin of doctors, especially when nurses and family had suggested his discharge was premature.

My experience is that many patients pressure hospital staff to discharge them too early. As well as this, the lifestyle of a patient in hospital and at home are typically very different, e.g. treatment for blood pressure when a patient is lying in a hospital bed may be inadequate when active at home.

Surgeons can only be in one place at a time, e.g. whilst doing private work they are not reducing public waiting lists, so maybe there is a case for more full-time public hospital surgeons, or separating the two roles. A start could be for private patients to be operated on in public hospitals, when opportunities arise. This may reduce downtime, due to surgeons changing locations, etc., and more effective use of public operating theatres, many of which are in use for about a quarter of the 168 hours available per week.

Alternatively, surgery in excellent facilities overseas, at a fraction of New Zealand costs, provides an opportunity for the government to subsidise patients to take advantage of this, even combining surgery with a holiday in a 'win-win' situation.

Sometimes improvement comes from looking outside an industry, e.g. in a paradigm shift the computer industry moved from huge expensive mainframes (affordable by big companies) to cheap, high volume personal computers accessible to most of the population.

Following this logic, why not devolve some of the work done by expensive specialists to others, such as pharmacists to screen for health issues like high blood pressure, as is done in the UK.

Starship Hospital in Auckland provides a service like the Australian Flying Doctor Service, transferring children to their 'centre of excellence.' Extending this idea to other specialties could be another means of reducing the strain on the supply of medical specialists, etc.

In 2013 Pharmac embarked on a public consultation program, seeking ideas for setting priorities for medicine expenditure. Along these lines, is it time for public discussion on challenging matters health professionals deal with every day? For instance, is someone too old to justify the high expense of treatment and should euthanasia be legalised?

Alternatively, in a real paradigm shift, do we need a greater focus on 'rewards for results' by paying health professionals (even health administrators) to keep us healthy, i.e. pay them a regular fee whilst we are healthy (and do not need medicines) and stop fees if this changes. A shift like this would increase the focus on patient lifestyle and their accountability, which could be ideal. One way to monitor progress would be to review the cause of all deaths, seeking ideas to improve lifestyle and reduce inappropriate treatment, adverse effects of medicines, etc. This could be anonymous, and firmly based on positive outcomes.

A 2013 news story featured a man so desperate he got his son to extract an aching tooth because he could not afford to pay a dentist. Given the poor state of dental health in New Zealand, the expense, and the fact that it constitutes a serious health risk factor, is it time for the government to subsidise treatment? Alternatively, tax concessions for those with health insurance, or develop systems like having a portion of an individual's taxes go into a personal fund to relieve pressure on the health system.

Over twenty years ago, the government withdrew tax deductibility for workers on wages who invested in work-related knowledge. Whilst people in business can claim such expenses, our citizens are our greatest asset, so why not reinstate this and extend it to those prepared to invest in health knowledge to achieve better health outcomes?

Social inequality is associated with many health and social problems.[175] Some of those who end up in prison actually need mental health treatment, so maybe we need more resources including safe, patient-friendly institutions. Radar detectors are a means by which the law can be flouted, increasing the chances of people becoming an injury statistic, so why not ban them?

Currently, some supplements are government subsidised. Recognising the value of complementary medicine, why not extend the list and allow pharmacists and complementary practitioners to prescribe them?

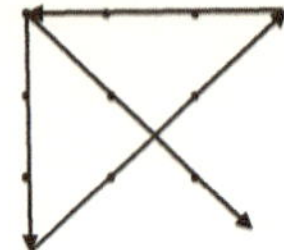

(The answer to the de Bono puzzle is apparent when you think 'outside the square.') By now, I am sure you have some good ideas of your own to add to the mix.

Transparency, trust and teamwork

In the television series *Undercover Boss*, chief executive officers (CEOs) who work undercover inside their organizations come to realise just how little they know about what their workers do. In many cases, they could not perform basic tasks, even though their management had set performance standards, poor working conditions etc. Most found staff had ideas to improve systems but these would only emerge with greater transparency and accountability. They realised a greater need for them and their management team to 'walk the walk' not just 'talk the talk.'

Not like the CEO of Telecom (France, 2012), who faces criminal charges associated with toxic work conditions and impossible performance targets, that led to over 30 suicides.

Some years ago I asked a Pharmac manager if any pharmacists on their staff worked in community pharmacy to understand what it was like to work with their rules and regulations. She suggested indignantly that I had no right to ask this question.

A newly employed health worker performed poorly at work, even though she had years of experience and had won academic awards. When reported to the authorities who had granted her qualification, they tried to wriggle out of any responsibility by saying, 'it was an employment issue, not one of competency.' Interestingly, most of her training was via correspondence, and her partner was qualified in the same field.

In 2011 bureaucrats decided prescriptions would be printed double-sided, to save paper. Whilst it sounds a good idea, what they failed to appreciate was the risk posed if pharmacists miss medicines when dispensing. To make matters worse, if an omission caused serious consequences, it is likely the system would let the pharmacist be the scapegoat. The idea was dropped and would not have got off the ground if they had taken the time to communicate with the profession, especially when the implementation process was poor and the importance of pharmacists being able to see all items when dispensing was not fully appreciated.

In 2003, community pharmacy owners like me had to renew their dispensing contracts, as happened every few years. The contract contained many unreasonable conditions, such as pharmacists being unable to claim payment for medicines (legally dispensed from a fax) until they received the original prescription from doctors, which could take weeks. I approached the CEO of my District Health Board about the issues and he said, "I do not have the power to negotiate conditions and if you do not sign the contract, I will have your prescription subsidy payments stopped." Under duress, I had to concede defeat.

Politicians, bureaucrats, professionals, private enterprise, the public and patients are all stakeholders in health, which is an expensive business. Just as a surgeon relies on a '**team**' (**t**ogether **e**verybody **a**chieves **m**ore) of professionals in an operating theatre, we need to ensure that stakeholders are part of a team.

Many decisions in life are emotion-based, yet are justified with logic. As we do not know what the future holds, all the planning in the world may count for nothing, if situations change, just as digital cameras have almost replaced film.

In light of this, effective organisations need to work together like the parts of a mechanical clock to achieve common goals, with empathy for all stakeholders and integrity, where high staff morale gives management the courage to make corrections along the way, without reservation. Hidden agendas, spin doctors, secrecy and bureaucratic inertia should play no role. Other key points to consider are:

- Feedback is an opportunity to improve processes.
- Systems reward those who raise issues that need addressing, especially when patient health and safety are at risk.
- Individuals are empowered to act professionally according to their code of practice.
- Staff acting in good faith are encouraged to report mistakes and learn from them without fear of punishment.

- It is easier to teach skilled technicians management than vice versa, so it makes sense to have more appropriately qualified employees in management and political roles.
- Public organisations need to be wary of sponsorship that compromises standards.
- Transparency counters conspiracy theories and lack of trust.

Helping each other

It is timely to recall the statement by Dr Andrew Moulden that changing the medical system to help people help themselves is the most important work we can do.

An example is an elderly woman who felt abandoned by the system. She was living alone and had a number of unresolved issues around mobility and chronic pain. In just a few minutes of chatting with her, one could see she was a sitting duck for a fall and fracture at a huge cost to the system. Like many other patients, this woman 'did not want to create a fuss.' If the system operated effectively, she would not need to

We all have varied skills and abilities, based on background, training and genes. Bear this in mind the next time you see anyone putting themselves above others. In fact, in *Outliers* Malcolm Gladwell highlights the work done by K. Ericsson in assessing that it takes 10,000 hours of practice to be top class in most activities, where opportunities along the way play a part that people put all down to 'natural talent.' This is a reminder of the huge amount of time, effort and money tax payers invest in training medical professionals.

Once I was with a group of friends wandering along a road, without a footpath. Realising the danger if a car approached from behind, I proposed that we walk on the right side of the road, to face oncoming traffic. A teacher in the group said that she had never heard of that idea. Knowing she taught new entrant children, I suggested she teach it to them. Sadly, she rebuffed the idea, saying, "I do not have the time, and anyway it's up to parents to do that." My response was, "How can that happen if parents don't know what they don't know, just like you didn't know this road safety rule?"

A documentary on AIDS (HIV) disease featured a 24-year-old woman who contracted it from a long-term relationship. She says, "Things would have been different if I'd been taught about this at school."

Out of ignorance, staff at a child centre in 2012 excluded a young child with AIDS. This highlights the ongoing need for authorities to keep a wide range of public health issues on the 'public radar' through brochures, advertisements, etc.

Our education system is costly, so it is reasonable to expect it to prioritise training in the essential life skills that employers and society want and that students need to survive. Priorities should include health and hygiene, sustainability, fruit and vegetable growing, healthy eating and personal relationships, all of which could provide a way to get spread messages to the community.

Years ago, my wife and I searched for a display-stand for health brochures in our pharmacy. Eventually we settled for a greeting-card stand, which worked well. Seeing the benefits, we suggest health authorities provide something similar for doctors' surgeries, pharmacies, council offices, etc. This should include regular checks to keep them updated.

Unfortunately, not everyone use resources available, e.g. in our pharmacy we dispensed many prescriptions for an angina spray over a 10-year period, yet to my knowledge, not one patient had been given the Heart Foundation's angina leaflet, nor had any asthmatic patients been given an 'action plan' (as issued by Pharmac) by their doctor.

Times have changed and we now see more people accessing online resources via smart phones, etc. The Ministry of Health's website [www.healthed.govt.nz] is a good place to start, with links to other resources.

Cures and prevention of disease

There are over one hundred different forms of arthritis (inflamed joints), with no cure for any of them. Imagine the time, effort and money poured into classifying the various forms. Whilst there has been some learning and benefit from this, a focus on real cures and prevention of disease would likely have led to more progress towards a remedy, rather than an increase in medicines (some of which have been recalled because of adverse effects, even death) and surgical techniques.

A classic story about cures involves researcher Dr R. Marshall in Perth, Western Australia many years ago. A BBC documentary, *Ulcer Wars* (1994) tells the story of how he suspected that an infection was causing certain stomach upsets and ulcers. To test his theory, he infected himself with the bacteria Helicobacter pylori. His research eventually led to treatment by short courses of antibiotics that often eliminate the bacteria and the problem. Until then, treatment was mainly lifelong acid-reducing medicines, which no doubt made good profits for the drug companies and suppliers.

Research now links the bacteria with stomach cancer, which is on the rise, affecting Caucasians in the USA, where over 50% of the population carries the bacteria, without visible signs of the disease. This information is very relevant to New Zealand that has a high rate of stomach cancer. [www.gicinz.org.nz]

The old adage 'an ounce (30g) of prevention is worth a pound (450g) of cure' makes sense, but marketing gurus say it is easier to sell the 'cure' or quick fix. Whilst the above story involves a real cure, a problem arises when health practitioners define cures as keeping patients on medicines for the rest of their lives, on a fee for service basis.

In light of this, many were horrified by a media report in June 2012 referring to a jump in the use of anti-depressant medicines for children. Pharmac has reduced medicine and distribution costs so dramatically, we are likely to see a continued focus on treating symptoms of disease with medicines, rather than finding real cures, or addressing other consequences, outside Pharmac's area of interest, including medicines polluting waterways and the medical costs of treating side effects and overdose.

Estimates suggest we spend much more on treatment than prevention, yet there is a four-fold return on investment when focused on the latter. 50% of New Zealanders have ongoing disease that accounts for a lot of our health costs. Thus illness provides a great deal of income for many health providers. Imagine how many would be out of a job if we were able to cure and eradicate most diseases right now. Thankfully future training for New Zealand doctors is to include more preventative medicine. Who knows, we may even see health practitioners issuing 'warrants of health' in the future.

As these ideas gain more attention, we will see a paradigm shift, with a greater focus on nutrition, lifestyle, disease prevention and real cures. This will happen when health administrators take a 'helicopter view' of things, to see the big picture and focus on installing a proverbial safety fence at the top of the cliff rather than an ambulance below to pick up the pieces.

These changes are likely to lead to significant financial savings, and a healthier and happier population, living longer. In fact, some medical conditions may even disappear, just as scurvy did, when Dr Lind worked out that a lack of vitamin C was the cause.

Responsibility

A study of 150,000 members of the public in the USA in 2000 found the following percentages engaging in healthy activities: non-smoking, 76%; healthy weight, 40%; five fruits and vegetables a day, 23%, and regular physical activity, 22%. Only 3% fulfilled *all* requirements.

This study highlights the challenges facing health authorities that spend vast amounts of money on health education, only to find messages ignored, possibly because the rewards from healthy living are often not immediate or apparent. Seriously consider your personal responsibility to your society exemplified by J. F. Kennedy when he said, "Ask not what your country can do for you, but what you can do for your country."

It seems most of us will take responsibility and act only if there is a reward, i.e. "What's in it for me?" A UK study appealed to vanity, telling participants they would appear more attractive within six weeks of eating more fruit and vegetables.

Ironically, some people are proud that they do not have a health provider, yet recognise the need to spend money maintaining their car. Take a lead from Mark Twain. "One of man's greatest regrets," he claimed, "is the things he didn't do."

So take responsibility for what you need to do before it is too late. Do not be like those in a state of blissful ignorance with an attitude of 'she'll be right, mate, it won't happen to me.' Don't do nothing, out of fear of what might be discovered. Early detection could make a big difference to the outcome.

Reflect how powerful the media is and how much damage can be done when it acts irresponsibly, reporting on subjects they know little about, yet commenting as if they do. Provocative unsubstantiated headlines and generalisations add to the confusion around health and well-being and can undermine the individual's confidence in the system. Remember, one study may not be enough to prove anything, e.g. a British surgeon's claims about autism links to the MMR vaccine attracted a great deal of media attention, yet the study was eventually found wanting and withdrawn, even though Wakefield stands by his research.

On the other hand, the media can be an influence for good. For example the heart surgeon Dr Oz is doing a great job with his television shows and website to help people take more responsibility for health [www.doctoroz.com]. With many guest presenters including complementary (CAM) practitioners, Dr Oz focuses on the big picture. *The Doctors* is a similar show [www.thedoctorstv.com]. It would be great if both were screened in prime time, with a message for conservative people to focus on the content, not the flamboyant style.

Aim to be like those who are passionate about taking pride in stepping up to the mark and taking responsibility. Most of us can achieve much more than we believe we can, often looking back to wonder why it took so long to act, especially when the solution to the problem turned out to be far easier than imagined. When it comes to health, many would like to take more responsibility, but do not know how to go about it. In some cases, health practitioners do not let them.

When doing market research for this book, some of those I questioned acknowledged that the responsibility of parenthood prompted them to accept a need for a greater focus on their health and that of their family.

When my wife and I took over our community pharmacy, we found patients knew little about their medical conditions and the medicines they took. We set about improving the situation and winning awards and are proud of what we did to change the culture, teaching them how to take more responsibility, even if much of the work was unpaid, because of how the system worked. Even today past customers tell us 'other pharmacies do not do what you did' and doctors say how their patients miss what we did for them. Maybe this book is an alternative.

Change

Just as there was a time when 'the umpire was always right,' tennis technology such as the Hawkeye system now confirms the 'facts', within a margin of error. In light of this, ideas about health will alter with time, ongoing research and changing attitudes. Whilst man has made significant progress towards winning the war on disease, we still have a long way to go.

What a shame we do not have access to nature's master plan, to show us how and why things work as they do to save us time, money and effort. Humanity has progressed out of a desire to experiment, grow and question. Sometimes change happens quickly, but it may also come slowly, like the banning of smoking in public places. We must be patient, as 'Rome was not built in a day.'

When considering change, it is helpful to understand the 'Pareto principle,' named after Italian economist, sociologist and philosopher Vilfredo Pareto, who, in 1906 observed that 80% of Italian land belonged to 20% of the population and that 20% of the pods in his garden contained 80% of the peas. The Pareto principle, also known as the 80/20 rule, states that for many events roughly 80% of the results come from 20% of the effort.

Apply this principle to your Action Plan and focus on what is not urgent, but important, instead of urgent stuff that is often not important.

My mission is to raise your awareness of the need to improve things, rather than bury your head in the sand. I trust this book stimulates further discussion amongst the public, bureaucrats, politicians, health professionals and patients alike, on how best to go forward into the future. As people come to the table with different perspectives and backgrounds, honest and respectful debate will be a valuable part of the change process.

Action

The message is to focus on taking action to improve things to lessen your chances of a premature (early) health crisis that could be brewing without warning. Do not be the person who needs a wake-up call like a heart attack to get active. Research often finds a gap between what people know they should do and what they actually commit to. Life is not a rehearsal and what you do today affects your tomorrow.

Hopefully you have identified areas you need to work on in your Action Plan to show you are serious about your health. Always consult your health providers for a diagnosis and to discuss the changes you are planning. Remember the old adage: 'Nothing happens if nothing happens.'

Continue to be grateful for your life and for all the people in it. Do not postpone important things, e.g. don't wait for your next check-up if you feel something is not right. Make an appointment and think of it as an investment in your health, not an unnecessary expense.

Some people do not know what they do not know, so may need help to recognise opportunities for action. Others feel like puppets on a string, or pawns in a system that is out of control, yet dictates what they can and cannot do.

Progress results when we recognise opportunities for improvement and act, instead of leaving it to someone else. For instance, the public protest against Cadbury substituting cocoa with palm oil in their chocolate caused the company to reverse its decision. Had it not been for 'people power' - in this case, the energy and enthusiasm of the instigators and the influence of social media - it is likely that nothing would have happened.

I encourage you to seize opportunities to improve our health system including talking to health professionals, administrators, District Health Board members, Pharmac or Members of Parliament. Remember there is strength in numbers and changes often take place only if a significant proportion of us act. It can be as simple as phoning a company to get health information about a product, just as I rang a high profile company to find out if dangerous trans-fatty acids (TFAs) were in their potato chips.

You will sometimes need to be persistent and patient, e.g. my call took ten minutes, talking to a customer service representative, then a supervisor, with neither able to give me an answer, or bother to arrange for someone to get back to me. If users of products and services are pro-active like this, eventually suppliers will get the message that change needs to take place, or they could lose business.

Other ways to act might include seeking information about how a product is produced, asking questions about what tests your doctor does at your next check-up, or requesting information from the local food store manager on the nutrient content of the produce you are considering buying.

If you work in the system, encourage managers to have a genuine 'open door' policy, to enable staff to fully engage with them about ideas to improve conditions and systems, backed up with incentives to make the effort worthwhile.

Staying on track

There are many ways to stay on track. Look for simple ways of preparing food and replace poor foods with better choices, e.g. replacing a white flour crust pizza with a stone-ground wholemeal flour base and using more vegetables and less cheese for the topping. Change from highly processed dips and chips to sliced vegetables dipped in hummus.[176] [177] Try replacing morning coffee with a healthy breakfast and morning tea with a glass of water instead of a coffee and muffin. Prepare a healthy lunch at home to take to work.

If hungry, try nuts and fresh fruit as snacks through the day. Carry a 'grateful stone' in your pocket to remind you how thankful you are for your life and to remind you of the need to continue working on your Action Plan. You do not have to replace food with food, so try replacing drinks and nibbles after work with meditation, a massage, music or exercise. Park away from work, walk and use the stairs instead of the lift. Play and sing along to your favourite music as you drive home to reduce stress.

Use all the tools you can: positive talk, sharing your goals, affirmation cards, social media, asking for help, keeping in touch with your coach, tracking your progress, mixing with positive, happy and healthy friends and colleagues. Emulate good role models and encourage and reward yourself for progress made. Also, strive to be a good example of health to the people in your life. You never know when some of your example will rub off.

The information contained here is intended to empower you to live a longer, healthier life by being proactive with your health and enjoying the results. Beware of quick fixes or magic bullets. This approach has limited benefits compared to a focus on the 'big picture,' akin to a fistful of cash, with each note representing strategies to improve your health which could save you money.

The key for healthcare in the future is to create a system that prioritises expenses appropriately, with all of us accountable and appreciative of the value of lateral thinking and transparency. We need to emphasise cures and the prevention of disease, rather than just treating symptoms with medicines and surgery. Of course, nothing happens if nothing happens, so we need to be open-minded and take action, all the while accepting responsibility and being a healthy example to those around us.

Remember, you are unique and need to get a professional diagnosis first. Because I believe we still have a way to go to understand health, be prepared for change. Be careful about what you believe, especially if taken from blanket media headlines that could easily misinform or confuse you, and be ready to do some research.

It is said that life is a journey and not a destination, so make this book the beginning of your journey to better health. What have you got to lose?

Feedback is an important part of this process. If you research a subject or have a story to tell, please let me know. I have a dream to create a forum of like-minded healthier people working together. Contact me through www.betterhealthforyou.co.nz, which has links to my Facebook page and Twitter account.

The best results in life come from having a plan, because vision without action is merely a dream. Fail to plan and you plan to fail. Think of the **four Ps**: **p**lanning **p**revents **p**oor **p**erformance. Doing the same thing repeatedly and expecting a different result is futile, like floundering around trying to work out how to use a new electronic gadget without reading the instructions.

Research suggests we are likely to forget three-quarters of new information if we do not move it into our long-term memory by revising it within a day, and on a regular basis.

The Action Plan form provides a tool to help you get results, so now it is up to you. Consider taking a photocopy to use as a working copy, or go to www.betterhealthforyou.co.nz to download a copy. Be sure to put it in a conspicuous place, to keep it on your radar, or carry a 'reminder stone' in your pocket. Along the way accept the things you cannot change (or change how you think about them.) Have the courage to change what you can and accept mistakes as lessons of wisdom, not to be repeated.

There are many tools available to help you make changes without relapsing, including, Maxwell Maltz's *Psycho-Cybernetics*[178] and Anthony Robbins *Awaken the Giant within.*[179] Here are some keys to achieving new goals:

- You cannot change what you do not acknowledge.
- Write down why you have not taken action yet, being scrupulously honest with yourself. Many hold back out of fear of failure (real or not) and do not appreciate anxiety about a challenge is normal for most of us. Do not let negative thoughts put you off.
- Beware of back-up plans that could give you an excuse for failure.
- Writing down goals and actions you need to take and sharing them with a coach and friends is important, as it is easy to say things and not follow through.
- Things become easier once you make a decision and act.
- Your emotions are powerful, so visualise your success and focus on reversing pain and pleasure, e.g. replace the pleasure of oversized pizzas and the pain of exercise with an image of the rewards of good health and fun activities and the pain if you do not change.

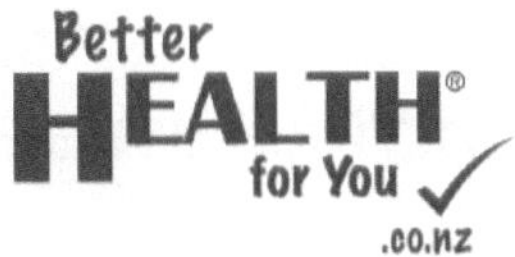

YOUR PERSONAL ACTION PLAN

Name ....

I rate my health as __ out of 10, and can see room for improvement.

My goals need to pass the **'Smart'** test, (i.e. **s**pecific, **m**easurable, **a**ction-based, **r**ealistic and **t**imeframed. I understand the Pareto principle (80/20), and that it takes *at least* 21 days to develop a habit.

My prioritised goals are as follows: (*Add another sheet if necessary.*)

....by   /   /

....by   /   /

....by   /   /

....by   /   /

....by   /   /

....by   /   /

....by   /   /

My Pledge
I will visualise, verbalise and act on my goals each day to achieve results.

My coach is ....

Email ....

Phone ....

Mobile ....

My coach will receive a copy of this plan within a week without fail and I will review this plan with my coach at least every three months to monitor progress and reset goals as necessary.

My signature ....   Date: ..../........../....

Coach's signature ....   Date: ..../........../....

Good luck and good health!

Denis Toovey was born in Perth, Western Australia and is married to Judy, a New Zealander. They have two children and six grandchildren. His interests include family, friends, woodturning, gardening, tennis, lawn bowls, reading and writing. After graduating as a pharmacist, he held a number of hospital management and clinical positions in Western Australia, working with administrators, doctors, nurses, patients and the Royal Flying Doctor Service. He also completed a Post-Graduate Diploma in Clinical Pharmacy.

In 1985 Denis moved his family to New Zealand, where he took up management roles that provided him with opportunities to introduce important innovations. He then worked for the Preferred Medicines Centre, advising doctors on cost-effective medicine usage. In 1995, he and his wife bought Avenue 12 Community Pharmacy, going on to win the prestigious Trustpower Customer Choice award three years in succession, in recognition of their excellent wholistic (big picture) customer service.

Following the introduction of three-months-at-once prescriptions, and finding themselves in a scenario that could not sustain their professionally focused, award-winning pharmacy, Denis and Judy closed their doors in November 2006.

Denis then tutored pharmacy assistants at the Bay of Plenty Polytechnic. Later, seeing an opportunity to bring quality health information to the general public (through touch-screen kiosks) he became national sales manager for Healthpoint Technologies.

Still with a passion to share what he has learned over 40 years, Denis set up www.betterhealthforyou.co.nz, runs health seminars, has written this book and is planning his next one on how we can have a more caring community.

REFERENCES

1   www.dietandcancerreport.org

2   Weill Dr A. M.D.

3   Readers Digest March 2011 pp32-37. www.readersdigest.co.nz

4   Roenneberg T. www.Health.com. May 2012

5   Whyte D. *Nature's Power Pack*. Huntly, NZ, Zestos Publishers, 2010

6   Goedeke Dr R. Clinical Nutritional Specialist. Auckland, New Zealand

7   Gurven M & Kaplan H. *Longevity among Hunter Gatherers.*

8   Staying Healthy Faculty, Harvard Medical School. January 23rd 2007

9   Bay of Plenty District Health Board

10   *LILAC (Life and Living in Advanced Age) Study in New Zealand.*

11   Buettner D. *Blue Zones.*

12   Goldacre Dr B. *Bad Science* p265. www.badscience.net.

13   *New Scientist,* 8 August 2009, p22

14   Repatriation General Hospital, www.auspharmlist.net.au/ebulletin

15   http://on.today.com/pWlo2Z

16   Gladwell M. *Blink.*

17   McCulloch EA & Till JE www.Wikipedia.org

18   D'Angelis Dr B. *Making Love Work Program.*

19   Maltz M. *Psycho-Cybernetics*. New York, Pocket Books. (1960)

20   *Bad Science* www.guardian.co.uk/commentisfree/2011/jun/17

21   Schwitzer G. *Bad Science*, p324

22   Esseltyn Dr *Prevent and Reverse Heart Disease*

23   Andrews Dr Z. Monash University, Australia

24   Ridker PM et al. 'Rosuvastatin to prevent vascular events in men and women with elevated C-reactive protein' *NEJM* 2008:359:2195

25   *New Scientist,* January 2011, p8

26   *Readers Digest,* May 2011, p74

27   *Journal of the American Medical Association* 2011 305(23):2448-55

28   Canfield J, Hansen M & Hewitt L. *The Power of Focus*. Vermil., 2000

29   *Readers Digest*. May 2011, p54

30   Hyperhealth Pro CD-ROM

31   American Diabetes Association. http://professional.diabetes.org

32   Morgan G. & Simmons G. *Healthcheque*
      http://garethsworld.com/shop/health-cheque/

33   *Int. J.l of Lower Extremity Wounds* March 2007 Vol 6, No. 1 pp18-21

34   *Scientific American*, December 2007

35   Tyler Moore M. *About Living with Diabetes*

36   Cabot Dr S. *Syndrome X*. New South Wales. WHAS Cobbitty, 2001.

37   *New Scientist*, January 2011 pp8-9

38   *Readers Digest*, May 2011 p40 www.readersdigest.co.nz

39   Colgan Dr M. *New Nutrition*.

40   Hyperhealth Pro CD-ROM

41   *Readers Digest Good Health Fact Book* www.readersdigest.co.nz

42   'Bugs from your gut to mine' *New Scientist* 22 Jan 2011, pp8-9

43   *New Scientist* January 2011 pp8-9

44   Law J. *Big Pharma*

45   Pelton R & LaValle B. *The Nutritional Cost of Prescription Drugs*. Morton Publish
      www.morton-pub.com

46   Hyperhealth Pro CD-ROM

47   Hyperhealth Pro CD-ROM

48   International Coenzyme Q10 Association. http://www.icqa.org/

49   www.mercola.com

50   www.transport.govt.nz

51   www.wikipedia.org

52   Pease A. *Questions are the Answer*.

53   Robbins A. *Awaken the Giant Within*. New York, Simon and Schuster

54   Cantu R. Professor of Neurosurgery, Boston, USA.

55   Roisen M. & Oz M. *You: the Smart Patient*.

56   Mayo Clinic USA (2009)

57   Cabot Dr S. *Raw Juices Can Save Your Life*. WHAS 2001 & SCB Camden NSW
      (2002)

58   Cabot Dr S. *The Liver Cleansing Diet*. www.liverdoctor.com

59   Moritz Dr A. *The Amazing Liver and Gallbladder Flush*.
      http://liverandgallbladderflush.com

60   Goldacre Dr B. *Bad Science*, p265. www.badscience.net.

61   Medsafe.www.medsafe.govt.nz

62   Theodosakis Dr J, Adderly B & Fox B. *The Arthritis Cure*. Pan Macmillan
      (1997)

63   Holt Dr S. & MacDonald, I. *Natural Remedies That Really Work.* Craig Potton (2010) www.naturalhealthreview.org

64   Law R. *Vitamins and Minerals, Herbs, Supplements.* (2002)

65   Hyperhealth Pro CD-ROM

66   Garcia A. & Koebnick, C. *et al.* (2008) www.ncbi.nlm.gov/pubmed/18028575 Long term strict raw food diet

67   Hyperhealth Pro CD-ROM

68   Harland J. Dr Hall Associates, UK. E-mail: jan.harland@harlandhall.co.uk

69   www.omega-3centre.com

70   Ridker PM *et al.* 'Rosuvastatin to prevent vascular events in men and women with elevated C-reactive protein' New England Jnl Med 2008: 359: 2195-207

71   Hyperhealth Pro CD-ROM

72   Price W. A. http://westonaprice.org

73   Wolcott W. *Metabolic Typing Diet.* New York, Broadway Books. (2002) www.metabolictypingonline.com

74   Hyperhealth Pro CD-ROM

75   Hyperhealth Pro CD-ROM

76   Oliver J. *Cook with Jamie.* (New York, Hyperion, 2007.)

77   USDA's National Organic Program www.amu.usda.gov

78   Chicago Institute of Food Science, 2009

79   Hyperhealth Pro CD-ROM

80   Szalavitz M. Psychology Today, July 2006 v39 i4 p54 (1) Sussex Inc.

81   Lassen A. & Ovesen L. *Nutrition and Food Science* July 95 n4 p8 (3)

82   Boutenko, V. *Green for Life.* North Atlantic www.rawfamily.com

83   *Supercharge Me! The Story of Jenna, a Certified 'Live Food Chef.'*

84   Campbell Dr T. *The China Study.* USA, Benbella Books (2005.)

85   National Institutes of Health (NIH) http://www.niehs.nih.gov

86   *Journal of the Science of Food and Agriculture*, v83, issue 14, pp1511

87   J Agric Food Chem v51, May 7, 2003, pp. 3029-34).

88   What's really in our food. www.TV3.co.nz

89   Laucke Flour Mills, South Australia www.laucke.com.au

90   New Zealand Food Safety Authority (NZFSA) www.nzfsa.govt.nz

91   Hyperhealth Pro CD-ROM

92   *The End of the Line* Documentary www.theendoftheline.com (2011)

93   *New Scientist*, 23 Mar 2011 p7

94   Hyperhealth Pro CD-ROM

95   www.cochrane.org.nz, www.cochranecollaboration.org

96   The Ministry of Health's Food and Nutrition Guidelines for Adults, http://www.health.govt.nz/

97   Wolf University of Nottingham

98   Katz Dr D. Yale-Griffith Prevention and Research Centre, USA

99   Green T & Venn B *et al.* 'Serum vitamin B12 concentrations and atrophic gastritis in older New Zealanders.' *Europ Jnl Clinical Nutrition* 2005:59:205-10

100   Scragg Prof R. University of Auckland, NZ www.fmhs.auckland.ac.nz

101   Borissova A. et al. 'The effect of vitamin D3 on insulin secretion and peripheral insulin sensitivity in type 2 diabetic patients; International Journal of Clinical Practice 2003, Vol. 57, No. 4, pp258

102   Osteoporosis New Zealand www.bones.org.nz

103   The relationship between boron and magnesium status and bone mineral density in the human: 1993 Seep's (3):291-6 United States Department of Agriculture, Grand Forks Human Nutrition Research Centre

104   Hunter I., *A strategy for the correction of boron deficiency in radiata pine plantations in NZ.* Forest Research Institute, Rotorua NZ

105   Hyperhealth Pro CD-ROM

106   Thomson C et al Dept. of Human, Nutrition., University of Otago, christine.thomson@stonebow.otaga.ac.nz

107   Walpole D. *Wot the Doc doesn't tell you.* Information booklet.

108   Finland Sympos, *Lancet,* July 2000. www.mtt.fi/met/pdf/met69.pdf

109   www.Wikipedia.org

110   New Zealand Heart Foundation. www.pickthetick.org.nz

111   www.activesmart.co.nz/nutrition/view/72

112   www.thecardiacclinic.co.nz

113   www.cochranecollaboration.com www.cochrane.org.nz

114   Warren B. www.BePure.co.nz

115   www.ausport.gov.au/ais/nutrition/supplements/

116   *Change One.* Readers Digest (2004). www.readersdigest.com.au

117   Bogusky A & Porter C. *The 9-Inch Diet.* http://www.livestrong.com

118   Hyperhealth Pro CD-ROM

119   Taubes G. *Why We Get Fat and What to Do About it.* Readers Digest (2012)

120   Kreitzman S et al. *American Jnl Clinical Nutr* 1992:56 292S-3S

121   Greene B. *The Best Life Diet Book*

122   PubMed http://www.ncbi.nlm.nih.gov/pubmed/21291433

123   Gluckman, Dr P., Government science advisor (2010+)

124 New England Journal of Medicine

125 Disease Free, Readers Digest 2011 www.readersdigest.co.nz

126 New Scientist June 2008.

127 Why are Thin People Not Fat, documentary, www.bbc.co.uk

128 Dubner S and Levitt S. *Freakonomics* www.freakonomics.com

129 Worth the Weight, Listener magazine April 23, 2011 page 16-21. www.diosgenes.org

130 Esseltyn CB Dr *Prevent Reverse Heart Disease*

131 'Cardiovascular quality and outcomes' *Circulation Journal* (2010)

132 Taubes G. *Why We Get Fat and What to Do About it*. Readers Digest

133 D'Adamo P Dr *Eat Right for Your Blood Type*. www.4yourtype.com

134 Dr Oz.com. *17-day diet* and *Resetting hormones*, with Dr M Moreno

135 *Change One*. Australia, Readers Digest. (2004)

136 Tolman D. www.dontolmaninternational.com

137 Fontana, St Louis Uni., USA and Italy. *New Scientist*, 29/5/10 p36

138 Food Hospital www.foodhospital.channel4.com

139 Gerson Institute, www.gerson.org/

140 What's really in our....' www.TV3.co.nz

141 www.tvnz.co.nz keyword food truck

142 Dow Dr M. *Diet Rehab*

143 Fletcher R & Fairfield K. 'Vitamins for chronic disease prevention in adults *JAMA* 2002:287:3127-3129

144 Dr Zheng Yee et al. *Europ, J. Cardiovascular Prevention & Rehabilitation* February 2008 vol. 15 no. 1 pp26-34

145 Jefferson: Manganese Super oxide Dismutase (MnSOD), Genetic Polymorphisms, Dietary Antioxidants, and Risk of Breast Cancer - Division of Molecular Epidemiology National Centre for Toxicological Research, Arkansas 72079 C. B. A.

146 Mares-Perlman JA. *The Body of Evidence to Support a Protective Role for Lutein and Zeaxanthin in Delaying Chronic Disease* (2002)

147 Norman I & Krinsky JT et al. 'Biologic mechanisms of the protective role of lutein and zeaxanthin in the eye' *Annual Review of Nutrition*

148 Mares JA, La Rowe T. & Blodi B. 'What vitamins should I take for my eyes?' *Arch Ophthalmol*

149 Depeint F. et al. 'Role of the B vitamin family on mitochondrial energy metabolism' *Chemico-Biological Interactions*. pp94-112 Vol.163, Issues 1-2, 27 October 2006

150 Bland Dr J. Biochemist and Prof of Chemistry

151 Whyte D. *Nature's Power Pack*. New Zealand, Zestos Pub. (2010)

152 Vitamin sprays www.vitamist.com

153 Littauer F. *Personality Plus*. Monarch Books, London NW7 (2000)

154 Brad Sugars www.actioncoach.com

155 www.healthcoaching.com

156 Wiseman R. www.invisiblegorilla.com

157 New Zealand Privacy Commission

158 'Colon cancer screening' *American Journal of Gastroenterology* 102.s2 (Sept 2007): p554 (1).

159 www.menshealthweek.co.nz

160 Dana-Farber Cancer Institute & Harvard Med. School, Boston USA

161 'What's really in our....' www.TV3.co.nz (2011)

162 'What's really in our....' www.TV3.co.nz (2011)

163 *Healthy Food Guide*. December 2008

164 Lifeline 0800 LIFELINE 0800-543354

165 www.breastcancerfund.org

166 www.safecosmetics.org

167 Neways www.neways.co.nz

168 Siemens www.Siemens.com

169 Readers Digest August 2010 p102

170 Hyperhealth Pro CD-ROM

171 Phelps, Prof. K. drkerrynphelps@acpmagazines.com.au

172 Holt, Dr S. (Miracle Pill) *Will you take the Polypill?*

173 Campbell Prof. T. et al. *30 minutes a Day to a Healthy Heart*. Readers Digest (2007)

174 Morgan G & Simmons G. *Healthcheque*. (2009) http://garethsworld.com/shop/health-cheque/

175 Wilkinson R & Pickett K. *The Spirit Level*. www.equalitytrust.org.uk

176 Campbell Prof T et al. *30 minutes a Day to a Healthy Heart*. Readers Digest (2007)

177 J. Nutrition 131: 3078S-3081S p2001

178 Maltz M. New York. *Psycho-Cybernetics* Pocket Books (1960)

179 Robbins A. *Awaken the Giant Within*. New York, Fireside/Simon & Schuster (1991)